MAKE UP

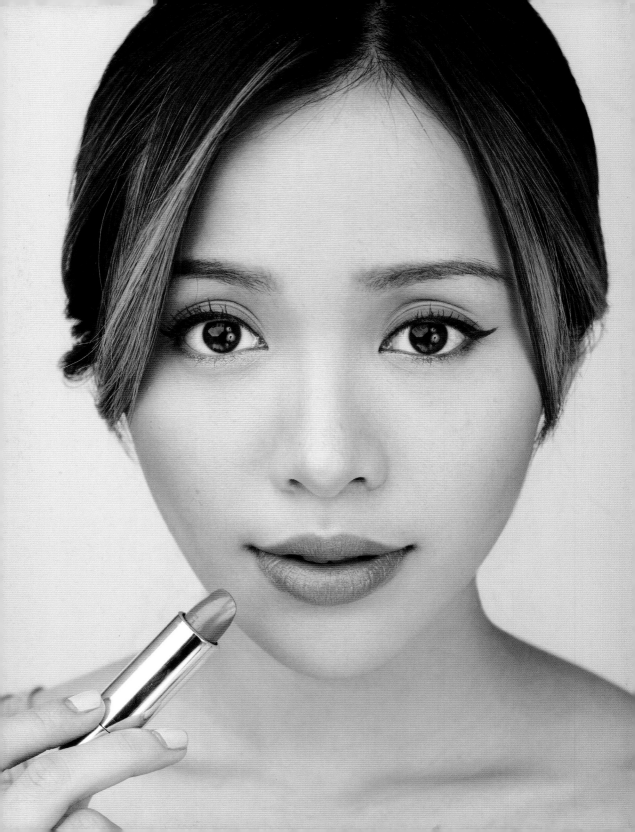

MAKE UP
MICHELLE PHAN

Your Life Guide to Beauty, Style,
and Success—Online and Off

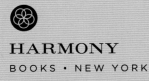

HARMONY
BOOKS · NEW YORK

HARMONY BOOKS is a registered trademark,
and the Circle colophon is a trademark of
Random House LLC.

All photographs by Josh Madson (hair by Octavio
Molina, styled by Flannery Underwood) with the
exception of those appearing courtesy of the
following:

Imagehub/Shutterstock: 68
Kerry Diamond: 18, 19
Roseanne Fama: 30, 31, 175
Linette Kim: 18, 19
Evan Jackson Leong: 155
Jimmy Jean Ngo: 25, 104
Jennifer Phan: 3, 6, 196
Flannery Underwood: 212
Wendy Wong: 24, 28, 79, 137, 150, 177, 186, 193, 198

Illustrations by Michelle Phan

Library of Congress Cataloging-in-Publication
Data

Phan, Michelle.
  Make up : your guide to beauty, style, and
success—online and off / Michelle Phan.
    1. Beauty, Personal. 2. Women—Conduct of
life. I. Title.
  RA776.98.P47 2014
  646.7'2—dc23
                          2013050664

ISBN 978-08041-3734-8
eISBN 978-08041-3735-5

PRINTED IN HONG KONG

Book design by Elizabeth Rendfleisch
Jacket design by Jessie Sayward Bright
Jacket photography by Mike Rosenthal

10 9 8 7 6 5 4 3 2 1

First Edition

*To my hero and the first person
who believed in me, my mother.*

*To my brother, Steve,
my first best friend.*

*To Christine, who gave me the
honor of being a big sister.*

*To Dom, who taught me how to
love unconditionally.*

*To all my close friends and family
who have given me a helping
hand on this journey.*

*And lastly, to my followers,
for giving me a chance
to see my dreams come true.*

Thank you.

CONTENTS

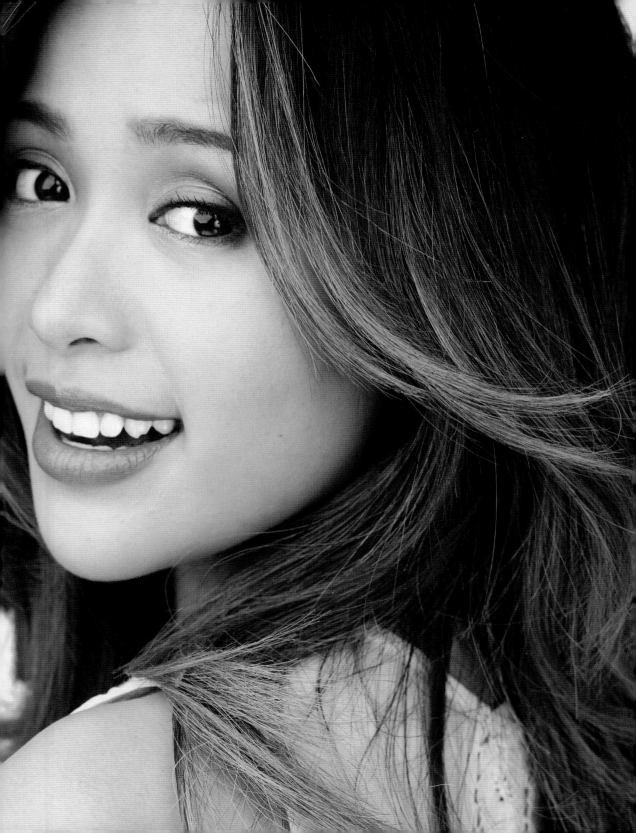

INTRODUCTION

Thank you for picking up *Make Up: Your Life Guide to Beauty, Style, and Success—Online and Off*! I am excited that you and I are about to take a journey through these chapters together. You might know me already, but for those of you who don't, here's a quick bio. I'm a former art student, self-taught makeup artist, and digital nerd who was lucky to see her hobby turn into a profession. Back in the early days of YouTube, I started posting beauty tutorials on a regular basis. A lot of people watched them, then a lot more. Within a short period of time, I had hundreds of millions of views and became the most-subscribed-to woman on YouTube. Making beauty tutorials became my full-time job. It was quite the twenty-first-century career and not the job I ever imagined having. From there, I've been on an incredible journey that's brought me around the globe and even seen the creation of my own makeup line, em. I've also launched a production company, a YouTube channel, and a beauty sample subscription service. I've gone from being a video-game-playing introvert to a CEO in a short period of time.

Creating a book is a new thing for me since I'm very much a creature of the Internet. When I found my calling online, my whole life changed. Through my videos and social media, I have been able to connect with people around the world. So why a book? Well, every day, on YouTube, Twitter, Facebook, Instagram—every digital platform that I'm on—I get asked questions about a huge range of topics. Everything from dating and making videos to dealing with acne and finding a job or an internship. I always wished there was a way I could answer all your questions. Now I can, through the pages of this book.

Books occupy an important place in my heart and my mind. When I was younger, before the Internet (yes, there was a time when the Internet as we know it didn't exist!), before Wikipedia, before blogs and websites and You-

Tube, books were my escape, my key to other worlds. My mom would drop me off at the local bookstore ("Don't worry, Mommy! I'll be fine," I would tell her) and I would stay there for hours, using the place like a library. I'd pore through books on art, makeup, and history and just get lost in the pages. I was in high school, often broke, sometimes bullied, and frequently misunderstood, and the bookstore was my refuge. To have my very own book is a dream come true. It would mean the world to me if this book helps you the way those books helped me years ago.

The past several years have been quite a roller-coaster ride of activity and opportunity for me, with many ups and downs and tons of life lessons. I've learned a lot the hard way, but I've also had the good fortune to meet so many inspiring, wonderful people and to be surrounded by loved ones, all of whom have helped me, taught me, and guided me through each stage. I've gained so much knowledge and I'm happy to be able to share that wisdom with you.

Nothing is more important to me than teaching, learning, and communicating. As I like to say, I live, I love, I teach, but most important, I learn. Let's have fun as you go through these pages. We'll dream, create, debate, laugh, and learn a lot about both of us. We're in this together. Sound good? Let's get started.

Good luck!

Love,

♡ Mish

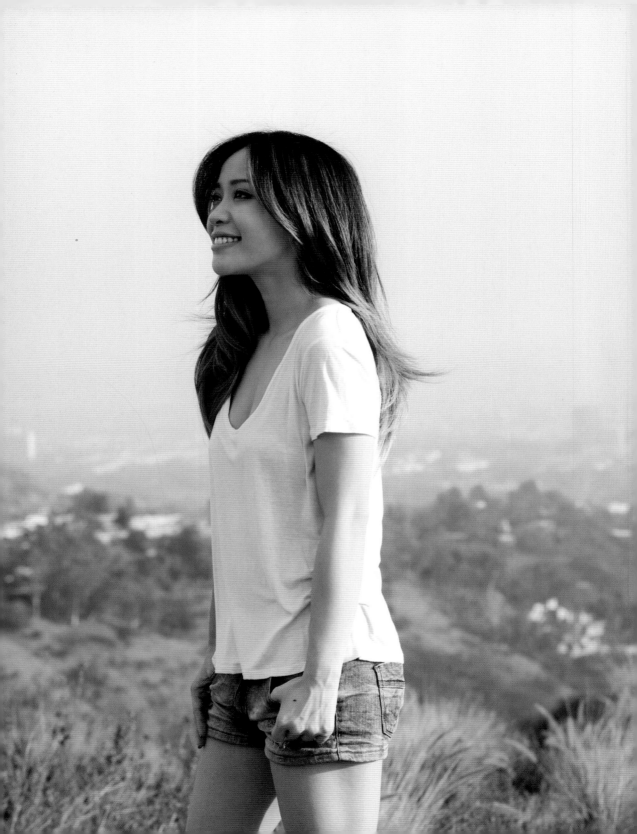

MY LIFE SO FAR, PART ONE

O ur stories are what make us unique. They are like fingerprints and snowflakes, and the stars in the Milky Way—none of them are the same. You, me, all of us are storytellers by nature. Sharing our stories makes us human and connects us to each other. It helps us to realize we aren't alone on this big, crazy planet we call home. What I'm about to tell you is not my life story, but my life-so-far story. It's the series of events that has helped make me the person I am right now, at this very moment.

Where should I start my life-so-far story? Let's go back several years and visit a little girl in a room filled with relatives. She's holding a crayon, her most treasured possession, and she's drawing. That little girl is me.

Even back then, I was always doing something creative. Remember phone books? The back section was filled with clean white sheets meant for note-taking, but I would rip out the blank pages and start drawing. The walls were another favorite canvas for my three-year-old self. My uncles would gently scold me—"Michelle, you can't draw on the walls"—as they scrubbed away my crayon scribbles. And then I would draw on the walls again the very next day. I didn't understand what I was doing, but I can see now that I had a strong natural desire to create.

My mom was wonderful about nurturing my artistic abilities. She would draw with me, and she taught me how to sketch faces. I'll never forget my first art lesson: I was four years old and we were sitting together in her room. It was a Sunday, her day off. She had a little calendar notebook that she filled with random things she needed to remember as well as poems that she wrote. On this day, she happened to be drawing a profile of a woman in her notebook. I was mesmerized as a face materialized with just a few strokes of her black pen. Suddenly and carefully, she drew this beautiful eye. I took a pen and started copying her, as she guided me along.

Perhaps that eye has been watching over me ever since.

My father can draw too, and I think he might be even better at it than my mom. He would sketch Teenage Mutant Ninja Turtles and Batman to entertain my brother, but he didn't draw for me. He knew I could do it by myself, and sure enough, in time, I was drawing Disney princesses and other magical characters. I saw my father recently, after a long time apart, and he said he knew, even when I was little, that I would grow up to be creative and independent.

MY PARENTS' STRUGGLE

My story really begins almost four decades ago in Vietnam, the country in Southeast Asia where my parents were born. My mother is from the countryside, in the south, and my father is from the north. Life back then was very hard for everyone because of the war. Both of my parents left their homeland with nothing and came to America as refugees. As difficult as my life was when I was younger, I was never tested the way my parents were. My mother remembers fleeing amid gunshots and jumping on a boat to escape. My father lived on a boat bound for Hong Kong for three months. Waves continually crashed against the vessel and the cold penetrated him to the bone. People were dying all around him. He prayed every night for a lighthouse to show the way toward land. Both of my parents wound up in the United States with few prospects but hopeful for a better life. They happened to have a chance encounter on a plane, fell in love, and ran away together.

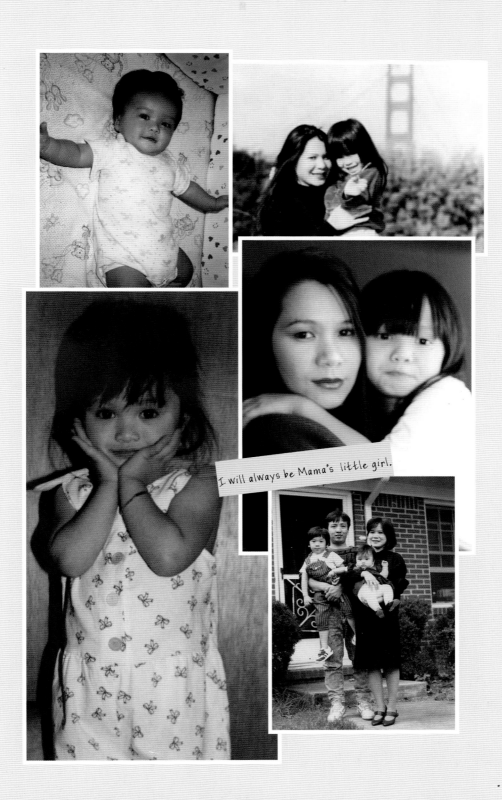

I will always be Mama's little girl.

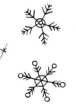

Years later, when my brother and I were born, my father gave us Vietnamese names that symbolized his struggle for freedom. My brother was christened Hai Dang, which means "lighthouse"—the very beacon my father prayed for when he was on the boat. And my name is Tuyet Bang, which translates as "snow that has exploded"—an avalanche. He wanted to name me after the powerful cold he felt for three months straight. "When you look at snow alone," he told me, "it's so delicate and beautiful. But when there is a lot of it, an accumulation, and something triggers it, it's an unstoppable force."

I didn't know the real meaning of my name until last year. Maybe that's a good thing. It's a great deal of responsibility to walk around with a name so meaningful to your parents.

Maybe you're wondering where the name Michelle came from. My parents wanted us to have American names in addition to our Vietnamese ones. Perhaps they thought it would be easier than growing up with the names Tuyet Bang and Hai Dang. My father, who was a construction worker specializing in flooring, was part of a crew renovating the home of a beautiful, wealthy woman in Boston. Exceptionally kind, she fed the workers and paid them extra wages. When he heard her name was Michelle, he tucked that in the back of his mind. Years later, as he and my mother were deciding what to call their new baby daughter, he knew that Michelle was the only option. He wanted me to grow up to be a generous, thoughtful woman like my namesake.

I was born in Boston, in what is now called St. Elizabeth's Medical Center, my parents' second child. We lived in that city for three months, then my parents decided we would have a chance at a better life in California. My father spent $600 on this jenky van and put a makeshift bed for my mother and brother and a crib for me in the back. Not quite the fancy baby car seats of today! There was no DVD player or satellite radio in this car. We were lucky the engine worked. The cross-country trip took four days. We arrived in downtown San Francisco, amid the street gangs and violence that were prevalent back then. My parents were scared and my mother wanted to return to Boston, but there was one problem: That car would never survive another three-thousand-mile trip. It was neither the first time nor the last that my parents would have to make the best of it.

WAY OUT WEST

We stayed in San Francisco for several years but moved around constantly to different houses and apartments. The last place we lived was in Oakland, in the Bay Area. It was tough on my brother and me. It's hard to develop social skills as a child with that much upheaval, not to mention what changing schools often does to your learning ability. I made one friend my entire time in California, and my poor brother failed first grade. Even at that young age, I felt very responsible for my family, but obviously I had no way to help them.

Our next destination was back across the country, to Tampa, Florida. My father thought the flooring business would be better there, but it wasn't. My mom, meanwhile, scraped together enough money to open a small nail salon, and went into business for herself. My father became a stay-at-home dad. Our little family was happy, but it was short-lived. My father returned to Boston to look for work, promising he would come back for us. I begged him not to leave, knowing deep down he would not be returning. "If you leave us," I told him, "I'll find you when I grow up." The next day I woke up and he was gone. Years later, he told me that he realized at that very moment I would be okay in life, no matter what happened.

I was right about my dad not returning. Our family was torn apart, never to get back together. Eventually my parents divorced and my mother remarried. I never got along with my stepfather, but the silver lining was the arrival of my beautiful little sister, for whom I am grateful every day. I was so happy to be a big sister.

Life at home was hard because of my family situation, and life at school was difficult too. You see, when we lived in Florida, it was the first time I felt truly different because of who I was. In California, everyone around me was Asian. I had felt self-conscious there because I was always the new girl, but it had nothing to do with my race, my color, or my heritage. Florida was different. Everyone in school was Caucasian, African American, or Hispanic, so as one of the few Asians, I got bullied. I would walk down the halls and the mean girls would say, "Ching chong, ching chong." The immature guys would get in my face and do Jackie Chan moves. Telling them that Jackie Chan was Chinese and that I was Vietnamese wouldn't have made any difference. All Asians were the same to them.

THE REAL ME

In middle school and high school, I tried so hard to blend in with different groups of people. I would put baby oil in my hair to make it shiny and wavy and get tan to blend in with the Hispanic girls. That didn't work. I asked some of my African American friends to braid my hair, thinking that would help me fit in. No surprise, that didn't work either. I was trying on different masks and different looks, but I was doing it for the wrong reasons. In time and through my videos, I would explore a range of identities to celebrate different facets of myself—and help others discover themselves in the process. But back then, I was doing it to hide the true me.

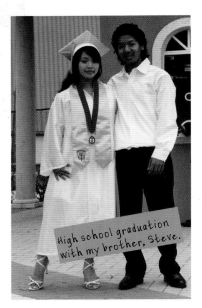

High school graduation with my brother, Steve.

How did I cope? By keeping to myself and staying busy. I am an introvert by nature, so it wasn't that hard. I taught myself how to play piano and how to paint. I wrote stories and drew comic books (which I still have because my mom kept them. Thanks, Mommy!). I could have easily fallen in with the wrong crowd if I didn't have my own little world.

By senior year, I was so tired of attempting to fit in that I stopped trying. I said to myself, "I don't care anymore. I just want to be myself. I'm an artist, I play video games, I'm a nerd, and I'm proud of it. I don't come from a wealthy background, but who cares?" And guess what? That is when I made a lot of friends. When I finally accepted myself, others accepted me. In my last year of high school, I felt like I got it.

MY DIGITAL ERA BEGINS

Today, we take the Internet for granted. Computers are everywhere. If you can't afford one, you still can access a computer at school or a public library or even an Apple Store.

Speaking of Apple, I was around fifteen years old when my family finally saved enough money, $600, to buy our first computer. We went to the store and looked at the few options we could afford, but of course I gravitated toward the Apple iMac G3. Remember that one? The egg shape with the jewel-toned panels? "It's different and it's cool," I said to my mother. "I like the design and I like the color." My mother shook her head no and pointed me back toward the cheaper options. But I just knew the iMac was a better computer. "Can we save a little bit more and get it?" I pleaded.

We headed home and started saving again.

When we finally got the iMac, I was so happy. It felt like we had this magical device in our midst that would let me explore the whole universe. The World Wide Web was still a new and novel thing at the time. I had heard about the Internet and saw it every once in a while at school and at the home of a girl I knew whose parents were well-off. She would go online and show me cool pictures of Sailor Moon and other anime characters and print out pictures of them. I was like, "What is this? It's amazing!" She gave me a tiny glimpse of this magical place and I wanted more. So when we had our first computer, I was always on it. I was a total computer hog.

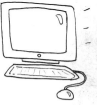

My mother didn't have rules for computer usage because it was so new. She wasn't alone; no one really knew what to make of it. It wasn't like TV. It was . . . different. "Mom, it's like the library," I would tell her, "but all in this computer." She didn't understand completely, but she liked the fact that the computer kept me home more.

In the beginning, I looked at a lot of anime stuff and discovered all of these blogs, which back then were mostly online diaries, a few of them written anonymously. The scene was so compelling that I wanted to join the conversation and start my own blog, focused on my artwork. I found a home for my blog on a site called Asian Avenue. It was just like it sounds—all Asians. Each week, Asian Avenue would spotlight a different member, who in turn would get tons of new followers. I wanted so badly to be member of the week, so I picked a name that I thought would help: Goddess of Asians. Can you believe? That's some name, right? It makes me laugh today. Looking back, I'm sure the people who visited weren't expecting to find a teenage girl's paintings and information on her favorite panda bear charity. But it worked. Soon enough I was member of the week and my following grew.

In a short period of time, I had this amazing group of followers and I started creating art just for them. It is every artist's dream to showcase her work and find an audience. It's why artists create.

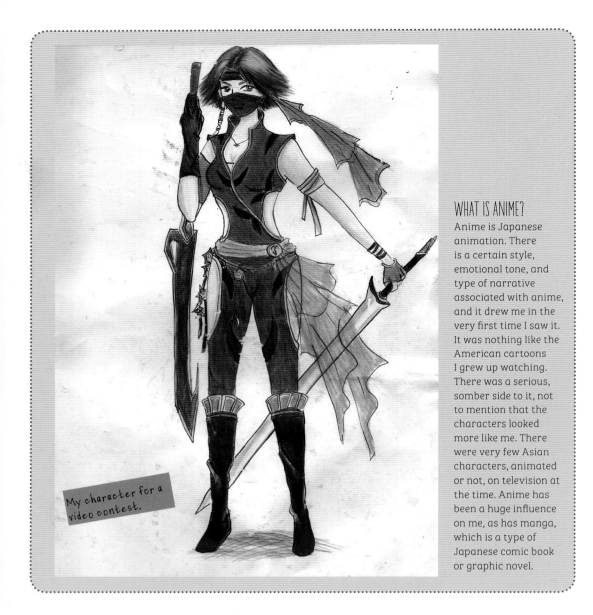

My character for a video contest.

WHAT IS ANIME?

Anime is Japanese animation. There is a certain style, emotional tone, and type of narrative associated with anime, and it drew me in the very first time I saw it. It was nothing like the American cartoons I grew up watching. There was a serious, somber side to it, not to mention that the characters looked more like me. There were very few Asian characters, animated or not, on television at the time. Anime has been a huge influence on me, as has manga, which is a type of Japanese comic book or graphic novel.

My paintings were inspired by different monthly themes I would choose. I guess you would call my style realism. I liked capturing real moments but interpreting them in my way, with different colors. I didn't come from a family that talked about art or visited museums, so I discovered this world on my own. One early favorite artist was the eccentric surrealist Salvador Dalí. There is a museum dedicated to him in St. Petersburg, Florida, which wasn't far from where I lived. You probably have seen pic-

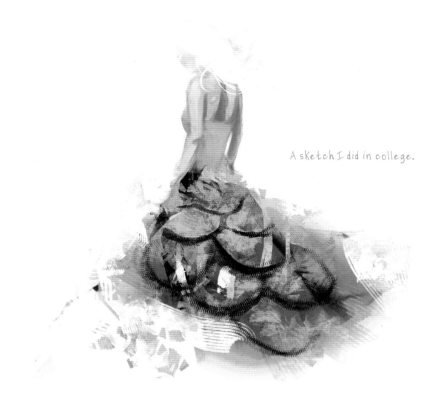

A sketch I did in college.

tures of Dalí, with his long, thin, curved mustache and crazy eyes. You've definitely seen his famous melting clocks from his painting *The Persistence of Memory*. He incorporates so much symbolism into a single painting that you could stare at the canvas for an hour and discover so many different things. Inspired by Dalí, I tried to incorporate symbolism into my work. Symbolism is everywhere if you just look for it.

The online communities back then were very positive. No bullying, no nasty comments. I could speak my mind freely in the popular chat rooms without being questioned or challenged because of my looks, where I came from, or my gender. No one in the offline world knew about my activities in this parallel universe. They would have written it off as strange.

> ## WHAT IS A SURREALIST?
> A surrealist is an artist who was part of the surrealism movement in the twentieth century. The surrealists' work blended dream-like visions with reality.

The next step for me, at the age of sixteen, was to join the hugely popular online platform called Xanga. I needed a better name than Goddess of Asians because Xanga was more personal. Michelle Phan was taken, so I decided to create a nickname for myself. "What's something original and cute and still me?" I thought. RiceBunny popped into my head because, well, I like rice and I was born in the Year of the Rabbit. That's all there was to it. I typed in the name and it was available. "Great," I said. "I'm

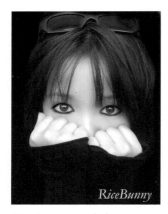

RiceBunny unveiled.

RiceBunny now." Who knew I'd be using that name for years, on all these platforms that had yet to be invented, like Twitter and YouTube?

My ambition was to be popular online because I wasn't popular in real life. In time, I became the most-subscribed-to female on Xanga; within two years, I had more than ten thousand subscribers. You might not think that is much by today's standards, but it was a lot back then; plus, Xanga was a very involved community. I focused on making my content as original as possible and each post I created received hundreds of comments. The subjects ranged from how-tos—how to paint, how to make a ninja mask, how to curl your hair—to entries about my art and my personal life. The latter entries, I'll confess, were embellished somewhat. The acceptance of the online community helped me grow as a person and an artist, but RiceBunny was a character, someone I aspired to be. She came from a happy family, she lived in a nice home, she had nice clothes. It was this persona I projected—and it was my online persona that people loved. I didn't expose the real me because I didn't think people would be interested. I wasn't comfortable in my own skin.

Everything changed in 2007, the year I made my first video, titled "Natural Looking Makeup Tutorial." Originally, it was meant to be a blog post. But right before I hit the "publish" button, I thought, "Makeup is so beautiful artistically and has so much movement. Let's make a video. Plus, you learn better watching than reading." I broke out my webcam, and with no idea what I was doing, I filmed the steps, edited everything, and added music and subtitles. I came up with my signature "Good luck" closing because I needed an outro. I uploaded the video and it took off. Soon enough, girls were requesting more videos—about smoky eyes, how to deal with acne, prom looks, you name it.

There was one problem. My videos didn't

> "Good luck" is how I end most of my videos. It's my way of encouraging the viewer to try what she (or he) just saw and letting her (or him) know that it's not always about skill. There's a little luck involved too, so experiment and have fun. You can always wash it all off and try again!

play that well on Xanga. I needed to move to a true video platform, so I started uploading on YouTube. In just one week, the natural-makeup tutorial received forty thousand views. Again, today's numbers are exponentially higher, but back then, this represented a lot of viewers. I had found my new home.

MIRACLES DO HAPPEN

I need to go back in time a bit. When I started posting videos, I was a student at the Ringling College of Art and Design in Sarasota, Florida. The road to my first semester was extremely bumpy, to say the least. My mother dreamed that I would work in the medical field, like many good moms do I guess, but my heart was set on art. I researched the best art colleges around and Ringling was the closest. I applied and got accepted almost immediately. But there was one big problem: tuition was $14,000, just for the first semester! For my family, that represented a fortune. We did not have the money, so I deferred admission for a semester, hoping for a miracle.

My mother, brother, and I were living together, pooling our money and trying to make ends meet. My mother worked double shifts at the nail salon, my brother had two jobs, and I was a hostess at a Thai-Chinese restaurant. Our credit was shaky, so student loans weren't an option. I prayed every day: "Dear God, I really want to go to Ringling. I have two months to find the money. Please help me find a way." Then one day, one of my mother's brothers from California came to town. He had done very well for himself in the construction business. He wanted to see where we lived, but my mother refused because she was embarrassed that we were living in one room with no furniture. My bed was a sleeping bag on the floor. Our clothing was in boxes. It looked very temporary, except we had lived like this for two years. None of my friends knew how I lived. My uncle insisted on coming over and he started crying when he saw what our situation was.

Back in California, he and my mother's other brothers and sisters got some money together and sent us a check for $10,000. They told us to use the money for rent and furniture, but my mother decided we would put it toward my tuition. We had saved $2,000, so that, plus the check, plus $2,000 on a credit card meant we had enough for me to start college.

That was the first miracle. The second one? Ringling decided that all incoming freshmen would receive a MacBook Pro laptop. I'll never forget going to school, grabbing a laptop, and hearing the sophomores complain about how unfair that was. I was supposed to be one of those sophomores! If I hadn't deferred, I wouldn't have gotten that computer. I could not have afforded to buy my own, not in a million years.

What was so miraculous about a computer? Well, that laptop, loaded with all its awesome programs, such as iMovie, iPhoto, and iTunes, and an internal camera, became the tool that let me truly express myself. I don't know if I could have started making videos without it. Everything I needed was contained right in that slim rectangle. In a way, it saved my life. It was my get-out-of-jail-free card. That computer was to me what the lighthouse was to my father. I will never part with it, even though I no longer use it.

After my first semester ended, I went back home. I wasn't working because my mother wanted me to focus on school. But it was clear she was killing herself to support us, working fifteen-hour shifts, breathing in all those chemicals at the nail salon. I didn't want that for her, so I started looking for a job. There was an opening at the Lancôme counter in the Dillard's department store at the local mall. It was a long shot because I had no retail experience, but I applied and was asked to come in for a test and an interview. I thought I did a good job, but two weeks rolled by and no one called. I knew if I could teach women how to apply their makeup, they would buy the products, and I told the woman who interviewed me as much. But it didn't matter. I wasn't what they were looking for.

A few days later, I made my first makeup video. Sometimes it is a blessing not to get what you want.

BACK TO SCHOOL

I worked really hard at school that first semester, so I received a scholarship and some grant money for my second semester. Here I was, leading a double life: beauty guru on YouTube and art school student. I kept my YouTube gig very, very quiet. No one on campus knew that I was a vlogger (that's a blogger who makes videos), and I liked it that way. But the videos were getting too popular and word got out. I was already a bit of a loner, so when people started making fun of me for the videos, I retreated even further. During breaks, the other students would be outside, smoking or getting snacks, and I was in the classroom, checking my YouTube channel, answering comments and messages. My professors certainly didn't understand. "Michelle and her little hobby." That's how they viewed it. They felt I was always online and needed to focus more on my studies and my painting.

Video requests were pouring in, so I knew something had clicked with the viewers and the people subscribing to my YouTube channel. All the money I had for art supplies was going toward makeup and video props. When I didn't have any money to buy white paint, the most basic of art supplies, it was clear I needed a job. So I started working at a really nice sushi restaurant, making $200 each weekend, enough for products and supplies and a little left over to send to my mother.

WHAT IS A BEAUTY GURU?

In the early days of YouTube, you had to pick a category for your videos. "Guru" was the option if you were making how-to videos. That's how all the girls doing beauty videos came to be known as beauty gurus. It wasn't a title we picked for ourselves, but it stuck.

Then a great thing happened: I started making money from my videos! The cash wasn't pouring in; it was only twenty cents a day. I was frugal, but no one in Florida can live on that. Still, it was something, and I was so excited. Where was the money coming from? Google, which owns YouTube, has a partner program in which content creators can earn a percentage of ad revenue. Slowly, the money increased to $20 a day. When I started making $200 a week, I gave notice at the sushi restaurant. "Are you crazy?" they asked. "You're leaving to make videos?" They reminded me that the economy had crashed and there weren't many options for someone my age with artistic aspirations. They told me they would keep the job open, but I urged them to give it to someone else.

I didn't want a safety net under me. I wanted to force myself to make this work.

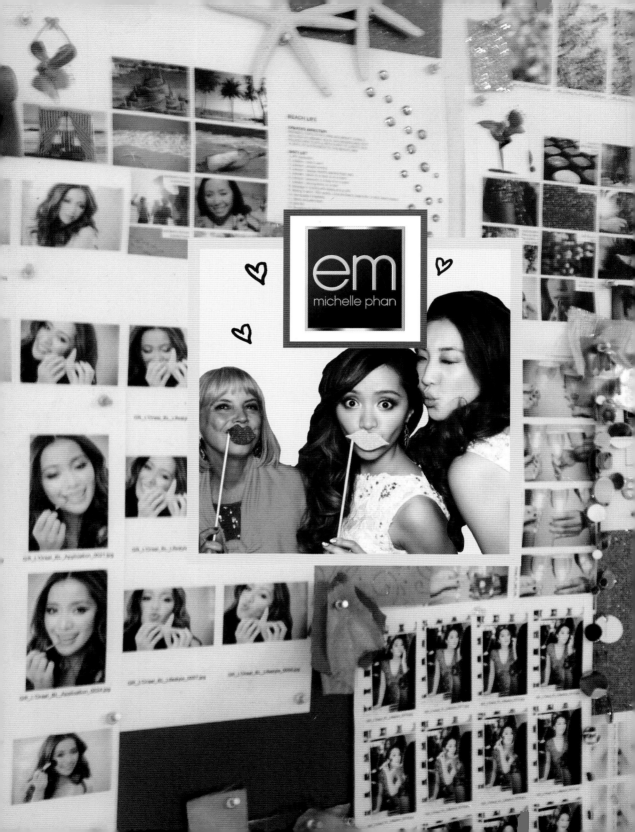

MY LIFE SO FAR, PART TWO

When you're a little girl and people ask what you want to be when you grow up, no one says beauty guru. Or vlogger. Or YouTube phenomenon. Here I was, all three of those things, part of this parallel universe that exists on the Internet and social media. I had gotten to this point by following my instinct to create, and by sharing and connecting with my audience. There was no guidebook or road map, or mentor to ask for career advice. I was on my own, with my very modern hobby that was quickly becoming a job. At the same time, I was still in college, still intent on pursuing the life of an artist.

I plunged into making videos. For months, I was completely focused on my YouTube channel and challenged myself to make every video better than the last. I wanted to differentiate what I was doing from the other beauty gurus' work. "What would I watch if I were that girl in front of the computer, instead of the girl on the screen?" I asked myself. My process was that simple. If I had a beauty big sister, what would I want from her?

My topics covered a wide range of material, from DIY (how to create a face mask using an egg, how to stretch out your ill-fitting shoes with ice, how to put some wave in your hair using paper-bag strips) to look-specific (prom, glasses, New Year's Eve, date night). I did skin care product reviews right in the drugstore aisle. I wanted to empower the viewer to try things for herself, to tap into her own creativity and experiment. My videos didn't require that you go out and buy specific things. Even when I used a certain product, it didn't mean you needed that exact item. You could use any pink lip gloss or any black mascara, for example. Glamorizing materialism wasn't my thing, which is why I didn't do "haul" videos, which involved nothing more than dumping your shopping bag on your bed and reviewing everything you had just bought—your haul. That kind of video was wildly popular at the time, and simple to produce, but I resisted. For me, the haul videos separated the "haves" from the "have-nots." Being a "have-not," I didn't want to celebrate that.

Instead, I wanted to celebrate making the most of what you have. That's how I have lived my life and that's what I wanted to prioritize.

Every single video broke the one million mark or came very, very close. I felt responsible to my audience and was grateful for every comment, suggestion, question, and view. It wasn't just the beauty-curious who were watching. More and more digital-savvy brands, from little beauty companies to major names in the tech world, were taking notice of the guru scene and started reaching out to many of us with various opportunities. I was a good businessperson from the start even though I was operating on instinct rather than lessons from a business class or book. I never sold myself or my audience short and took the easy money. From the start, I tried hard to stay true to my values and the messages I wanted to convey.

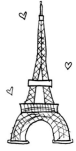

THE PARIS CONNECTION

One day, in the time it took to read an e-mail, my life changed. I was checking my YouTube inbox when I noticed something from Lancôme, of all brands. Curious, I clicked it open and sure enough, it was from a representative in the New York office of the French beauty brand. It seemed legit, so I wrote back. It was legit all right. Lancôme wanted to fly me to New York so I could meet with the boss of the U.S. division. I was so shocked I had to read the e-mail a few times.

It turns out the Lancôme executives were big fans of my videos. They had first noticed me when I used a Lancôme concealer in "Airplane Makeup Tutorial," a video where I did my makeup squeezed between two other passengers and recorded it on my laptop. It was a fun, simple video—certainly not one of my more artistic or complicated efforts. Still, it caught their eye.

I had to cut class to fly to New York, but it's not every day that the biggest luxury beauty brand in the world wants to meet with you. I obsessed over my outfit and my makeup—of course!—and put on my game face. We had a nice lunch and a great meeting and I went back home. We continued to talk and I continued to make my videos and go to school, until one day they popped the question. "Would you like to be Lancôme's official video makeup artist?"

How many ways are there to say yes?

At the time, no other brand in the entire beauty industry had a video makeup artist, let alone a brand as prestigious as Lancôme. Actually, most beauty brands weren't even making videos at all. Brands understood the Internet, and most of them had websites and were selling their products online, but social media was very new and the biggest names in beauty and fashion were taking baby steps, if any steps at all, in that direction. For many of them, social media meant putting too much power in the hands of the consumer. Brands liked having control.

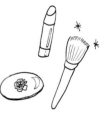

So what did this new job mean? It meant I would be a spokesperson of sorts for Lancôme. Me, the person who was turned down for the job at the Lancôme counter in Dillard's. Remember that story?

I was already using Lancôme products and loved the glamour and heritage behind the brand. Plus Lancôme was willing to give me control over the look, feel, and content of the videos I would make, which was a very important factor for me. I said yes and we embarked on a groundbreaking partnership. It was a first in so many ways, for the industry and for beauty gurus. But most important for me, it was recognition of what I had been quietly doing down in Florida for the past few years. Empowering women through makeup meant everything to me. Now, with Lancôme's help, I could reach more women than I ever imagined, online and off.

When I made a video announcing the news, most of my "subbies" (those who subscribe to my YouTube channel) were thrilled, but some people criticized me in the comments section. Usually, I would feel bad about any kind of criticism, but this time I didn't. "I'm having my Cinderella moment and you can't take that away from me," I thought. It was amazing to represent this brand and be part of beauty history. At the time, I was the only Asian spokesmodel for Lancôme and the first Vietnamese spokesmodel. There was much to be proud of. Besides, a girl needs to pay the bills! I wasn't this doll living inside the computer. I was a real person supporting herself.

As exciting as everything was, there was more to come. Things truly exploded thanks to American *Vogue* Editor in Chief Anna Wintour, always a big fan of what's new and next. *Vogue* did a story titled "Logged On." It stated: "Every generation in fashion has its force to be reckoned with, but this group is the first of its kind. It blogs about style and is making a global industry sit up and take notice." I was featured, along with well-known bloggers Garance Doré, Bryanboy, Todd Selby, and Hanneli Mustaparta.

People did sit up and take notice. Lancôme was bombarded with interview requests for me from media outlets around the world, from local newspapers in Canada and Poland to CNN and the *New York Times.*

My responsibilities for Lancôme increased and I began representing the brand not just in the United States but around the world. I was flying up

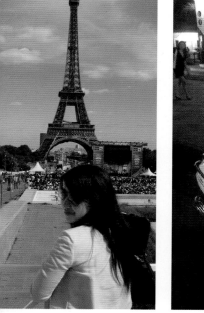
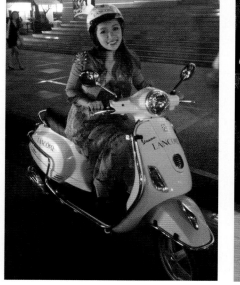
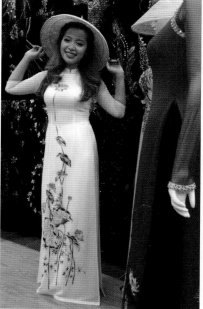

to New York frequently and had to make a very difficult decision about my studies. My family had scrimped and struggled to get me into art school. I was a junior now and had my senior year ahead of me, but I was missing too much school. My life was changing in ways I could never have imagined. With so much opportunity at my doorstep, I decided to take a year off from school. I truly thought I would return and finish my degree, but I never went back.

In a way, I exchanged art school for the world's best internship. My Lancôme job never felt like work; instead, it was an amazing opportunity to learn how the beauty industry operates and to see the world. The Lancôme team took me on my first trip to Paris. If you are a romantic like me, you can't help but fall in love with that city. We went to Beijing and Hong Kong too. We did photo shoots with all the major magazines, including *Vogue China*, and took part in a big press event introducing me to the Chinese media. It was exciting to meet all the beauty editors and see how cool and stylish they were. I was surprised to see they didn't wear much makeup, but they were all obsessed with skin care and nail art! And great shoes.

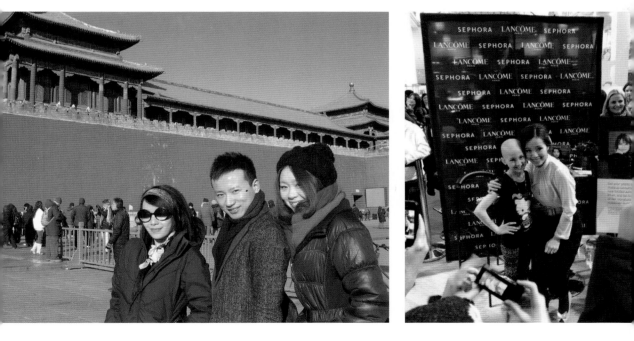

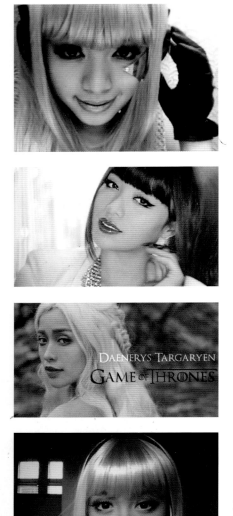

DAENERYS TARGARYEN
GAME OF THRONES

FROM GAGA TO ANGELINA JOLIE

Lancôme wasn't my full-time job, even though it took up a lot of my time and attention. Less than half of what I posted on YouTube was for Lancôme, so I still had to produce my other videos. I continued to push myself creatively. As much as everyone loved my straightforward tutorials, the biggest reaction came from my dramatic transformations. I wanted those videos to be like mini-movies for my viewers. I turned myself into a sexy vampire, a Tim Burton character, Sailor Moon (my anime heroine!), and everybody's favorite, Lady Gaga. How did I do this? Well, if you haven't watched the videos, you need to! There were no special effects involved. Just makeup—sometimes lots of it—plus really good props.

The Lady Gaga videos got a huge amount of attention, although I'm not sure if Lady Gaga herself ever watched them. If she did, I hope she liked what she saw. The videos were made with love and admiration for her talent, her creativity, and her message.

Despite the massive number of views for my Gaga tutorials, they weren't my most watched videos. Do you know which one is the most popular? It's "Barbie Transformation Tutorial," a lively and very pink video I filmed for Halloween 2009.

Speaking of Halloween, that holiday is like the Olympics for beauty gurus. Each year, the videos get more and more extreme as YouTubers undergo transformations worthy of the best science fiction and horror movies. Body painting, face prosthetics, elaborate wigs, you name it. It's all there each October. You should check it out if you haven't already. My Halloween looks aren't as dramatic as some, but they're still fun. I've morphed myself into everything from a zombie Barbie

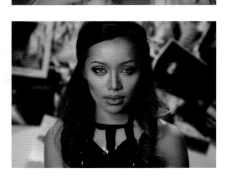

to Snow White to Princess Jasmine from *Aladdin* to Angelina Jolie. I could never fool Brad Pitt, but I think you'd be surprised what you can achieve with some contouring makeup, lip liner, and colored contact lenses!

To make all of this happen, I was constantly reinvesting my money into more makeup, props, wardrobe, and wigs; better camera equipment; and editing software. I wanted to create videos with a longer shelf life than the average beauty tutorial. If you watched them in ten years, I wanted them to feel as fresh and as relevant as the day I uploaded them to YouTube.

STILL TRYING TO FIT IN

I was definitely an anomaly in the beauty industry. I was a makeup artist, but not a traditional one, meaning I didn't do makeup on other people— I did it on myself. I worked with a big makeup artist agency in New York for a short time and learned from the experience, but it was hard when they booked me for traditional jobs, such as working on photo shoots and backstage at fashion shows. My agency was trying to shoehorn me into what they knew and I was having an identity crisis. I just wanted to be myself, but what did that even mean?

Not much scares me, but my first-ever backstage experience, at the Michael Kors fall 2010 show, was terrifying. Everybody knows Michael Kors, right? He's one of the most famous designers in the world and his runway show is major! Here's how the whole backstage thing works: The designer hires a top makeup artist to create

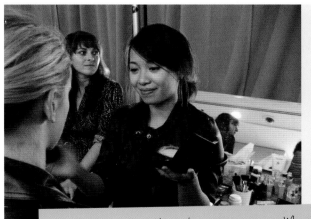

Smiling helped me get through my nervousness. When you're scared, a smile will always give you courage.

the beauty "look" for the show and the artist brings his or her team to re-create that look on all the models. It's crazy backstage because there are dozens of shows taking place each day during Fashion Week, and the models run from show to show, sometimes arriving late. So you have the entire makeup team, the hair team, all the models running in, racks and racks of clothing, the designer and his or her employees, plus all the press: bloggers with their iPhones, newspaper photographers with their big cameras, and TV crews with their booms and video equipment, all jostling to get a quote or a great picture. As each model arrives, she rushes to an empty chair and quickly gets her makeup done. Quick is the operative word—and I'm the opposite of quick. That's the nice thing about videos. I can make them at my own pace. But in fashion, it's fast, fast, fast!

Michael's lead makeup artist was Dick Page, one of the most important and talented artists in the industry, and the models in his show happened to be the biggest supermodels around. These were the A-list faces, the ones you see in the pages of *Vogue* and *Harper's Bazaar*, such as Karlie Kloss, Chanel Iman, and Liu Wen.

The night before the show, I fell asleep, scared about what the next day would bring. Suddenly, I started dreaming. There was a tall man wearing a black T-shirt and jeans and holding makeup brushes standing with his back to me in a room with a mirrored makeup table. He turned around and it was Kevyn Aucoin, the greatest makeup artist ever and one of my heroes. "Kevyn, I'm really scared," I said. "I have a show I have to work at and I'm not sure what to do." "Look. Here are some tips," he said, and showed me how to apply concealer and powder to a model's face. "You're going to do fine. Don't worry," he told me. "Good luck."

I woke up and burst into tears, out of shock and relief I guess.

Because of him, I went backstage and I wasn't scared. But I was slow. I managed to do one model; the other artists did three each. One of the show producers could see I wasn't very seasoned, so she gave me some cotton balls and acetone and told me to remove everyone's nail polish. "Great. I got the newbie job," I thought. "I've totally failed at this one."

The experience made me realize I never wanted to do another backstage show. "It's not for me," I said. The pace was too fast and I didn't like doing makeup on models. It was a hard decision to come to because some of the

WHO IS KEVYN AUCOIN?

Kevyn is a legendary makeup artist who died way too soon at the age of forty. His bestselling books, *Making Faces* and *Face Forward*, were a huge inspiration to me and countless other makeup artists. He was the king of the transformation and one of the first artists to do red carpet, magazine covers, advertising, and fashion editorial. Very few artists do all four.

most talented makeup artists in the world do fashion shows. Would I be considered less of a makeup artist if I skipped this entire category of the business?

It didn't matter. I needed to be true to my talents and myself. Lesson learned.

GOOGLE COMES CALLING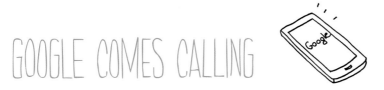

I have had a good relationship with Google from the beginning of my YouTube career. The executives there refer to me as one of their "children." In turn, I always refer to the company as "Mother Google." They are proud I created my brand without showing off body parts or doing anything vulgar. Often, videos that go viral are of the raunchy, sexy, or gross-out-comedy variety. But that was never my thing. I proved you could build a following with wholesome content.

Still, I was surprised when Google came to me with a proposal to start my own production company. Google wanted me to create additional content for YouTube and was willing to give me the support to get it off the ground. Of the other YouTubers that Google approached, I was the only beauty guru. Despite all the views, comments, likes, and buzz, I still frequently second-guessed myself and questioned whether I was making the right kind of videos. (But that's normal, isn't it? No one is sure of herself 100 percent of the time.) For me, the offer helped validate what I had been doing all these years.

The message that came through was to trust my instincts. Following my gut had gotten me this far, after all. But I was about to learn it takes more than instinct to be a success.

As part of the deal, my production company would develop original programming for a new YouTube channel. The channel was called FAWN. I liked the play on my last name, plus it lent itself to a great acronym: For All Women Network. Instead of starring in all of the videos myself, I thought it would be fun to use this opportunity to collaborate with other YouTubers. So I brought in several of the top beauty gurus, including Bethany Mota, Andrea's Choice, Promise Phan, Chriselle Lim, and Jessica Harlow.

FAWN also featured newer talent, helping to build an audience for up-and-coming YouTubers Theodore Leaf, Daven Mayeda, Charis Lincoln, and Rachel Talbott, among others.

Sounds easy enough, right? Great name, great concept, great talent, funding in place. Well, not exactly. The first year was a shaky one. I made some hires that didn't work out and I was learning—quickly—how to think big-picture. It's one thing to be singularly focused on your own channel, where you are the director, producer, camera operator, editor, and talent all rolled into one. It's a big leap from that to head of a network. Granted, FAWN wasn't ABC or HBO, but it was my own smaller version.

Google, to its credit, let us find our way and put a lot of trust in us. The company wanted to be kept in the loop but didn't get involved in our decision making. My team and I tried lots of different things; some worked, some didn't. We did a travel show called *Wanderlust* and visited Rome and New Zealand. Other shows focused on careers and took viewers behind the scenes of the fashion industry, where we spent time with luminaries such as editor Eva Chen and supermodel Coco Rocha. I also interviewed Grammy Award–winning artist Nelly Furtado and international style icon Dita Von Teese.

Thanks to Google, I got a crash course in production and learned a great deal about leadership, business development, and budgets. The first twelve months were like a year spent working toward a virtual MBA. FAWN was exclusive to YouTube for the first year, but now we're allowed to work with other media outlets and expand our scope of activities. So stay tuned. We're in the process of transforming FAWN from a production company to a media company, and I know great things will come of it.

THE ROAD TO IPSY

When I was younger, I used to hang out at my mother's nail salon all the time. It was a small place, but she made enough money to pay the bills and help our family get by. The salon was a sanctuary to me. I would watch *Gilligan's Island* on the TV in the back, do my homework, and eavesdrop on the conversations out front. When I was finished with my studies, I would read all the beauty and fashion magazines lying around. *Allure* was my favorite because it had these beauty and skin care how-to cards that you could tear out and save. I collected them like other kids collected baseball cards. But the real treasure was when the magazine contained a sample glued to an advertisement or a scent strip for some new fragrance. I tested and smelled everything.

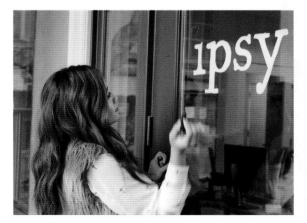

As a high school student, I didn't have money for makeup, so I would shop from the returns bin at the local drugstore. Everything was super cheap and you just had to wipe the product off, scrape away a layer or two, or sharpen the pencils a few times and they were as good as new. I managed to put together a small makeup collection for just seventy-five cents per item. Yes, in many cases it was used product, but that was okay. Who knew that one day Chanel and Yves Saint Laurent would send me bags overflowing with their products? I certainly wasn't dreaming that big as a teenager!

Fast-forward several years to Thailand and my first visit to the country. I was shopping with a friend and we stumbled upon this kiosk loaded with samples for sale, all packaged in little clear plastic bags. These weren't junky samples from random brands. These were full-size samples from the best names—La Mer, SK-II, Lancôme, etc. Girls were going crazy over them. I asked my friend why they would pay for samples and she explained that in Asia, you can't return beauty products, even unopened ones, so you only buy things you've sampled. "That's so smart," I thought. "I would love to do something like this in the States."

A few years later, I had a meeting with an Internet executive to discuss a few opportunities. I told him one of my dreams was to create a beauty subscription service that offered full-size samples. He wasn't very impressed, as other subscription services already existed, so I told him about Thailand and how much girls love real samples.

The goods offered by some of the other services were things you could get for free on your own, I explained. I wanted quality samples, not just trial-size foil packets with one application of lotion or conditioner. Let's create something really exciting, I told him. In a way, I was paying tribute to my younger self, the girl looking for samples in the pages of a magazine and buying other people's unwanted products.

That's how MyGlam came to be. It was a beauty-sample subscription service that you could join online. For a fee, you would receive a different makeup bag each month, filled with a range of beauty-product samples. I wanted it to be the best subscription service out there and to build a community of people sharing tips and recommendations.

However, the first few months were rocky. We sold one thousand bags our first day in business. Then in just ten days we sold out of bags entirely. The whole MyGlam team put all the boxes together ourselves. We were small and scrappy. We didn't have a logistics or packaging company. We continued to grow and grow, hitting twenty thousand bags, then thirty thousand. Once, the product offering was supplemented with some foil-packet samples, something I said I would never do. I was upset when I found out, but it was too late. The bags were already released. It was a good lesson for me: Make sure the people around you know what your non-negotiables are. This was one of them!

I knew instantly that we would lose customers because of it, and we did. Subscribers were mad at me—rightfully so, because my name was on this project. I collected the team and said we needed to start over. No foil samples, ever. Only deluxe and full-size. We had to work with the best brands and we had to make each bag we offered fit a real theme: beach beauty, prom night, red carpet ready. The subscribers should be able to create a full look. We went back to the drawing board and started doing things differently. One thing still nagged at me—the name. I never liked MyGlam, but we had needed to register something and I was tapped for ideas. So MyGlam it was. As part of the rebranding, we decided to find a new name. Not everyone wants to be glamorous, after all! Sometimes you want to be sexy, sporty, cute, preppy, or classy—or a combination of all that. So ipsy was born. And ipsy is anything you want it to be.

We owned up to our mistakes and moved on.

I'm happy to report that ipsy is now one of the most successful beauty subscription services around. The company is based in San Mateo, California, and we're still in start-up mode in terms of our mentality and size. I'm proud of the ipsy team and I'm thrilled that we have a roster of YouTube beauty all-stars who help pick our products and create ipsy how-to videos.

THE NEW GENERATION

Since I started making beauty videos back in 2007, the online beauty community has grown exponentially. However, it remains very fragmented. Was there a way, I wondered, to bring everyone, all the vloggers, bloggers, and Instagrammers, together? Despite our being a fairly tight-knit community—though, of course, there are some rivalries—most of us had never met in person. How could we make this "community" a real community?

The ipsy team was frequently invited to participate in beauty conferences as a sponsor, but none of the opportunities felt right. I've been to a

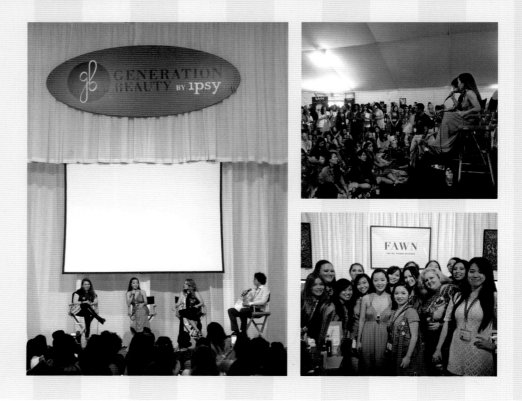

We are celebrating a new generation of women who are empowered.

lot of these events and many of them were disorganized and boring. So I thought, why not host our own, have it focused on digital beauty, and amp up the excitement level? We could invite all the beauty content creators plus the most-loved brands, but only the ones that understood the digital scene. (You'd be surprised, but many brands just don't get it—still, to this day!) With that, Generation Beauty was born. The goal? To be the best beauty conference ever.

As you can imagine, getting Generation Beauty organized was like planning a giant wedding. For the space, we selected L.A. Live, the entertainment complex where the Los Angeles Lakers play, and we had a giant pink carpet made for the entrance. We planned seminars, workshops, and parties. Tickets went on sale and sold quickly. We flew in the top beauty stylists and gurus from around the country to lead the various panels. The big day arrived and it was beautiful, with more than twelve hundred people in attendance and more than twenty brands participating. The sessions were very productive, as experts shared everything from makeup techniques to business lessons. Our live Instagram feed was on fire. We handed out tons of amazing products. And since you can't live on lipstick alone, we had L.A.'s best food trucks lined up outside so everyone could experience the city's famous food truck scene.

As with everything, lessons were learned. The ipsy team did a great job executing the particulars, but in retrospect, we should have given ourselves more time. It was stressful getting everything planned and completed with the deadlines we set. Now my goal for Generation Beauty is to become the best conference for beauty bloggers and digital content creators around the world. We will come together, from every country, not as competitors, but as sisters and friends—to bond, network, and learn.

THE BIRTH OF EM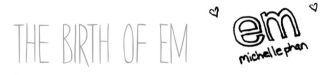

Back at Lancôme, I was about to get some unexpected news. The president of Lancôme's U.S. division asked me to go to dinner with a few other executives to catch up. "Uh-oh," I thought. I hadn't heard from him in a while, so this might not have been good. En route to Nobu, the Japanese restaurant in midtown New York where they were taking me, I felt pretty anxious. We all sat down and ordered, and then he started talking. "It's been great working with you," he said, making it seem like the end was near. In my head, I was telling myself, "Okay. If they fire you, just say thank you, hold it in, and be gracious. Make sure not to cry or be upset." The whole thing unfolded in slow motion.

So when the president said, "We'd like for you to have your own makeup line," I stared at him in disbelief. This was my dream come true, but had he really just said those words?

The makeup line he was proposing wouldn't be part of Lancôme. It would be a new brand, created from scratch, under the umbrella of L'Oréal, the biggest beauty company in the world. So many thoughts flooded my head and I was excited, eager, and anxious all at once. I felt like Cinderella when her fairy godmother appeared and turned the pumpkin into a gilded carriage.

The project was top secret. I wasn't supposed to tell that many people, but I did call my mother when I got home. At the dinner, one of the executives said this brand was a white canvas for me. I took this as a sign, because I always tell people life is like a blank canvas. What you put on the canvas is up to you.

The initiative was given the code name Project Sister and L'Oréal put together a small team to work on the launch. I managed to juggle all of my responsibilities: making videos for Lancôme, YouTube, and FAWN; overseeing ipsy and making videos there too; and working with the Project Sister group on every single detail. It was hard and a lot of work, but it was thrilling at the same time. The Project Sister team flew to Paris to meet with the world's leading expert on mascara brushes and we sat through countless packaging and product-development briefings. For a beauty nerd like me, this was heaven. The core team and I spent so much time together we became like family.

My brand needed a proper name. I loved the word *em*, which seemed perfect in every way. It literally was a reflection of *me*. In Vietnamese, *em* is a term of affection meaning "little sister," "girlfriend," or "sweetheart."

We officially launched in August 2013. The September issue of *Vogue*, traditionally the biggest fashion magazine of the year and a huge deal in publishing circles, hit newsstands with a story about em. Actress Jennifer Lawrence was on the cover and to the bottom right was a cover line that read: "Phan-Tastic! Beauty Blogger Michelle Phan's 700 Million Views." This

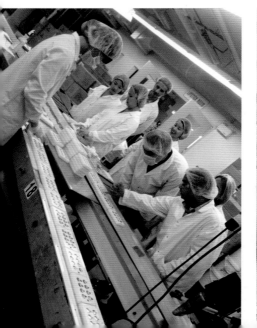

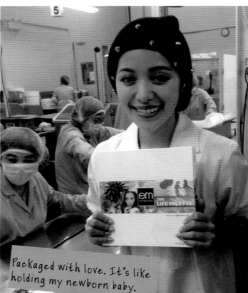

Packaged with love. It's like holding my newborn baby.

was a very humbling moment. *Vogue* Editor in Chief Anna Wintour and her beauty director, Sarah Brown, always believed in me, even when other magazines wanted nothing to do with me.

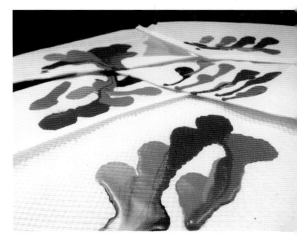

To celebrate the launch, L'Oréal threw a big party for everyone who had worked on em, plus my family and friends. Once onstage, I dedicated em to my mother, who was in the audience with my sister. "I am a reflection of my mother and she is a reflection of me," I said.

If my mother hadn't been so fearless all those years ago, if she hadn't worked tirelessly to take care of her family, none of this would have happened. All she ever wanted was a better life for herself and her family. She is my hero.

WHAT'S NEXT

As you might imagine, I've gained a great deal of wisdom through all of these opportunities and experiences. I never expected to be where I am—not in my wildest dreams. I even received an honorary Doctorate of Arts degree from Ringling College. Being my own boss and having multiple companies was never my goal. I even told a friend once that I'd rather just work for someone and go home at the end of the day so I could watch my favorite TV shows and play my favorite video games. That's where my head was less than a decade ago!

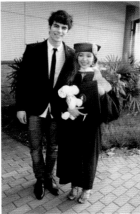

For whatever divine reason, I found myself on this road, with no compass or map—or Google Map, for that matter! As I journeyed along, I had faith that it would lead me somewhere good—I just didn't know exactly where. Now I'd like to help you on your journey. The pages ahead are filled with lots of information, all of it practical, a lot of it fun. Not only will we find your path together, but I'll help you look, feel, and be your best as we travel along.

Let's get started. And, of course, good luck!

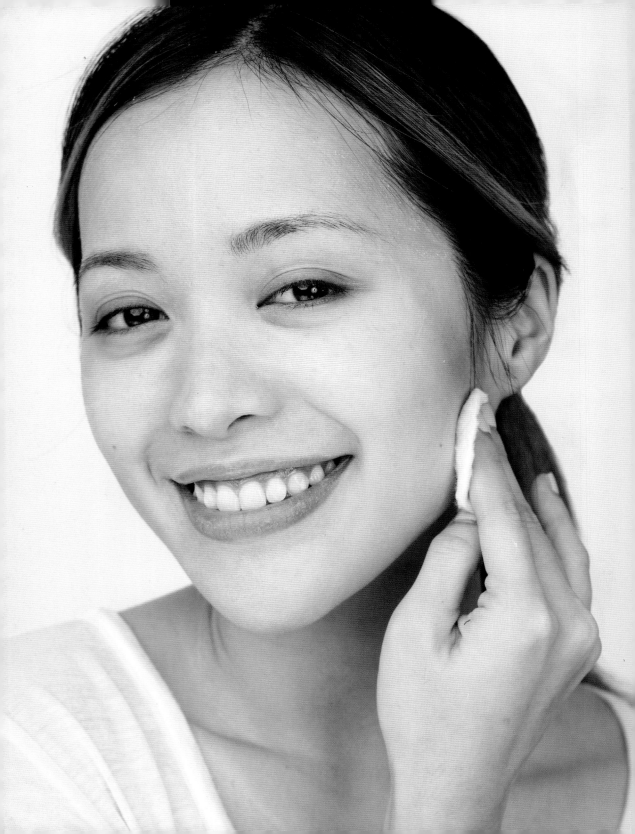

SKIN CARE SAVVY

Perfect skin? I don't want you to get hung up on chasing perfect skin. It's an idealized state that very few people can achieve. You either have perfect skin thanks to genetics or you don't—or perhaps you have a very expensive dermatologist helping you out! Most models and actresses don't have perfect skin, although they appear to. They just happen to be the beneficiaries of expertly applied makeup, retouching, and great lighting. If you met them in person, you might be surprised.

So why even read this chapter if perfect skin is unattainable? Well, I want you to have the best skin possible and chances are you can improve the current state of your skin. There are steps each of us can take to ensure that our skin is in optimal condition and we'll discuss what those steps are. So perfect skin? No. But better skin? Absolutely.

UNDERSTAND YOUR SKIN TYPE

The first thing you need to do is figure out your skin type. (This will come in handy when we discuss makeup in the next chapter.)

There are four basic skin types:

Normal
Dry
Oily
Combination

The first three mean exactly what they sound like. Normal is normal, dry is dry, oily is oily. If you don't have any skin issues, your skin type is most likely normal and you are very lucky! If your skin feels tight, crinkly, or even itchy, it's dry. If your skin feels greasy and is very shiny, you probably have oily skin.

The last category, combination, means you can't fit your skin type into one neat box. Sometimes it's normal and sometimes it's dry, for example. Or perhaps your T-zone is oily and the rest of your face is normal. It could be any combination. I generally have normal skin, but it skews a bit oily.

A WORD ABOUT ACNE

Acne is not a skin type. You can experience acne no matter what your skin type happens to be. It used to be thought that only teenagers with oily skin and bad diets got acne, but today we know acne is a disease of the skin and affects a wide range of people of various ages. There are ways to deal with this condition, and the first thing to remember is not to blame yourself. Acne is often hereditary, but that doesn't mean we need to live with it. We'll talk more about acne in the sections ahead and discuss what you can do to fight it and lessen its impact on your life and your skin.

YOUR SKIN CARE ROUTINE

Once you understand your skin type, it's time to think about your skin care routine. This is simply the steps you follow to take care of your skin and the products you use. Hopefully you have a routine already. If not, I'll help you develop one! And if you do have a routine, I'll help you refine it.

I am fanatical about skin care, so my routine is fairly elaborate. I believe good skin takes work. When I went to Asia for the first time, I was so excited because I met women even more skin care obsessed than I am. Some of them use as many as a dozen skin care products each day! That is dedication. My routine isn't that complicated, but it still involves several steps and one or two products for each step. When I follow my routine to a tee, I wake up with hydrated, moisturized, and bouncy skin. It took me some time and experimentation to find out what worked best for me. I promise that paying attention to your routine and finding what is right for you will pay off for your complexion.

STEP ONE: CLEANSING

Most people overcleanse their skin. Have you ever washed your face with soap and gotten that tight, squeaky-clean feeling? That is not a good thing! You've stripped your skin of essential moisture. I cleanse my face twice a day, but never with soap. At night, I use eye makeup remover to take off everything around my eyes—shadow, liner, and mascara—and then wash the rest of my face with a drugstore cleanser that foams slightly. In the morning, I dampen a cotton pad with water and refresh my skin with it. That's it.

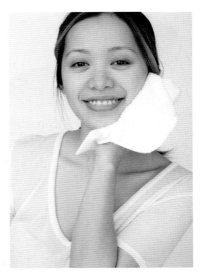

If your skin type is dry, I would swap the foaming cleanser for a non-foaming creamy cleanser. This will remove makeup and clean your skin without stripping it.

If your skin type is oily, use a gentle foaming cleanser morning and night. Remember, you don't want that tight feeling after you wash. Just a clean feeling.

CLEANSER VERSUS SOAP

Is one better than the other? In general, I find most soaps too harsh for facial skin. Of course, there are some on the market designed just for the face, but even those can be too strong. I know some people can't imagine having clean skin without a good soaping down, but it is possible!

Cleansers are liquidy or creamy and come in a container or a tube. There are two varieties: cream cleansers and foaming cleansers. But it's not that

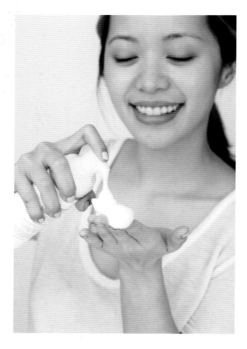

simple. Within the cream cleanser category, some get slightly foamy, while some don't and are purely creamy. And within the foaming cleansers, you get some that foam slightly, and some that are very foamy and stripping, making them not that different from bar soap. The wording on the packaging of some cleansers can be unclear, so they don't really explain what you're getting.

Confused? Sorry. It is slightly confusing. But once you find the right cleanser for you, this will be easier and your skin will be all the better for it. Look for sample-size cleansers at the drugstore you can try before buying the full-size option. If you're at a department store beauty counter, ask for samples. Don't be shy. That's why companies make samples. They hope you'll like the product enough to come back and spend your money on a full-size version.

REMOVING YOUR MAKEUP

You should never, ever go to bed without removing your makeup. It's no different from brushing your teeth. Both are activities that should be nightly routines in your life. (I won't even bring up flossing, but hopefully you floss at night too!) As I mentioned, makeup removal is a two-step process for me. First, I use an oil-based eye makeup remover because you need a very targeted product to gently break down makeup such as mascara and liner. Your basic cleanser doesn't have what it takes, whereas the oil in the remover will help break up the product.

Saturate a cotton pad with remover and press it against your eyelid and/or lashes. Leave it on for a few seconds so the product can do its job, then wipe the makeup away. Don't try to do your eyelid and lashes all in one swoop. Do a section at a time.

Use a cotton pad for safe eye makeup removal!

Don't use cotton balls to remove your eye makeup. They're not effective at the job and will leave wispy threads in your eyelashes. Don't ever rub or tug at the area around your eyes. The skin there is very thin, so you need to be gentle.

Next, I wash my entire face with my cleanser. Your cleanser

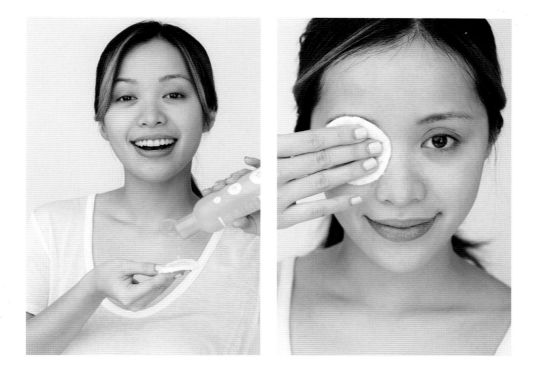

should be enough to remove the rest of your makeup. If you find that you still have makeup residue on your face, try using makeup remover wipes or towelettes before your cleanser. The combination of eye makeup remover, wipes, and cleanser should get off every last bit of makeup.

"Lazy Girl" Makeup Removal

You come home late from a date, a party, work, whatever. You're super tired. You know what it's like—we've all had those nights. All you want is to put your head on your pillow. The last thing you want to do is take off your makeup and wash your face. But please—do not go to sleep with your makeup on! That's the worst thing you can do for your skin. At the very least, use makeup remover wipes or towelettes and give your face a quick once-over. Try not to tug or rub too much when taking off your eye makeup with the wipes. If you buy wipes that both hydrate and remove makeup, you can skip moisturizer and go straight to bed. Sweet dreams!

> *Can I use makeup remover wipes for my eye makeup?*
> You can, but you might find they aren't saturated enough to remove your mascara. A targeted product is a better idea.

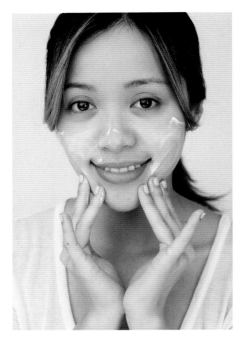

STEP TWO: SUN PROTECTION

I think it's fair to say that I'm obsessed with sun protection. Everyone knows that sun exposure causes wrinkles, so the earlier you start protecting your skin, the better. There are so many great sunscreens on the market that you really don't have an excuse for not using one. Formulas used to be heavy and greasy, but there are lightweight and sheer versions today that you will barely notice on your skin.

I like to apply my sunscreen in the morning, right after I've cleansed my skin. I do this before applying any other products, like serum or moisturizer. I believe that your skin needs to absorb the sunscreen for proper protection. This just happens to be my personal preference. If you want to put sunscreen over your products, that's fine. I use a minimum of SPF 35 and apply it to my face, neck, and chest. Your chest is very prone to sun damage because the skin there is so delicate. It's easy to forget to apply sunscreen there, but try to make that one of your daily skin care habits too.

Every time I see my mother, I'm reminded why it's good to use sunscreen. She's been using it for decades and doesn't have any wrinkles!

DON'T FORGET YOUR HANDS!

I always apply sunscreen to the backs of my hands. I split my time between L.A. and New York, and when I'm in L.A., I drive all the time. Your hands are exposed to a lot of sun when they're on the steering wheel. Your hands tend to be the first place where signs of aging appear, so some vigilance when you're younger will pay off.

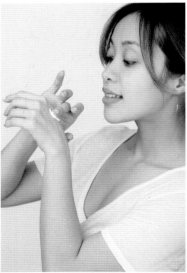

STEP THREE: RETINOID CREAM

I'm a big fan of retinoids, a special category of skin care product. These are creams derived from vitamin A and renowned for their ability to boost collagen production and smooth fine lines. Retin-A is the most famous retinoid around. You need a prescription for the most effective retinoids and they can be expensive, although you only use a tiny bit at a time. They're powerful products, so using more doesn't mean it will be more effective!

Every evening, I apply a retinoid cream to my nasolabial folds (the "lines" that run from outside your nose to the corners of your mouth), my forehead, and my crow's feet (the little lines that radiate from the corners of your eyes). I do it to prevent wrinkles. It's not that I'm against aging; I'm just looking to slow it down. This is one of the steps I'm taking.

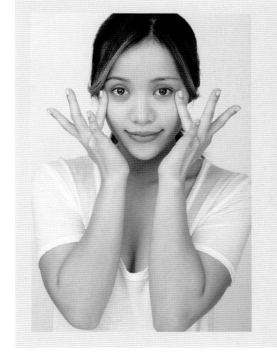

So why doesn't everyone use retinoids? Well, some people find their skin is too sensitive. You need to be religious about sun protection when you're using retinoids because they can make your skin more sensitive to sunlight. There's also the cost and the hassle of getting a prescription from your doctor.

If you're trying retinoids for the first time, don't use your product daily. Start by applying it every few days and let your skin get used to the product. You should discuss all of this in advance with the doctor giving you the prescription.

Want an over-the-counter version? Look for a retinol product. Perhaps you've seen this word before. You'll find serums, night creams, face masks, moisturizers, and more with retinol as the key ingredient. You won't experience the same dramatic effects as you would with a retinoid, as retinol is a less powerful version. But it's definitely less expensive and easier to acquire. You still need to be smart about sun protection though, retinoid or retinol!

I started using a retinol moisturizer when I was seventeen. I liked to raid my mother's beauty bag and use her products. When I hit my midtwenties, I upgraded from retinol to retinoids. Really, it's up to your discretion as to when you start using these products. Retinol is gentler and less abrasive than retinoids, so if you've never tried this supercharged vitamin A ingredient, take a baby step and use a product that contains retinol first.

STEP FOUR: SERUM

Serums are another category of skin care that might be new to you. Basically, they are supercharged creams that provide a range of treatment benefits. You wear them alone or under your moisturizer. I apply serum all over my face, chest, and neck as part of my a.m. and p.m. routines. In the morning, I apply serum on top of my sunscreen. In the evening, I apply it after using my retinoid cream.

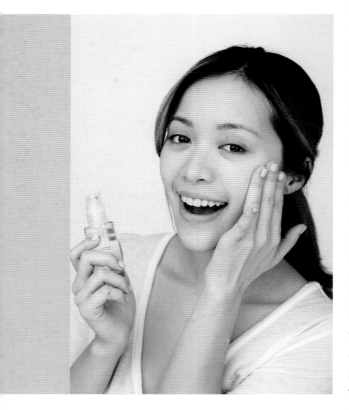

There are a few factors to consider when choosing your serum. First, what is your budget? There are serums at every price point. Next, figure out the treatment benefits you want. You can find serums that help fight acne, lighten dark spots, boost collagen, hydrate—you name it. I prefer ones with wrinkle-fighting ingredients plus antioxidants, because my job can be stressful and I live in a polluted area. This way, I get antiaging benefits and I give nutrients back to my skin.

I started using serums when I was in my late teens because of the lack of sleep and stress I got from school! Think of serums as coffee. They wake up the skin and give it life! Without the jittery effect, of course.

STEP FIVE: MOISTURIZER AND EYE CREAM

After serum, I apply eye cream. A lot of people think they can skip this step, but I feel that paying attention to the area around your eyes will pay off in the long run. The skin there is delicate and prone to wrinkling, so why not take care of it? On top of that, it's sometimes the first area on your face to wrinkle, so a bit of prevention is wise. I use a small amount and pat it under each eye using my ring finger (which happens to be the most delicate finger!). Anything left over is applied to my lids.

Next, I apply my moisturizer. I prefer gel-based moisturizers to creams because they are lighter and feel nicer under foundation and makeup. Although I layer several products on my face, I don't like the feeling of lots of layers, so the gel texture is perfect.

You want to consider your skin type and skin care needs when choosing a moisturizer. If you have oily skin, you'll want something lightweight. (Yes, even oily skin needs moisturizer.) Dry skin? Look for something richer and creamier. Normal skin? You'll want something in between that hydrates nicely. Budget is another consideration. If you're using sunscreen and serum first (and perhaps a retinoid cream), you don't need a fancy moisturizer. You'll find that similar to serums, moisturizers can range in price from affordable to outrageous!

I apply moisturizer all over my face, chest, and neck, morning and night, right over my serum. It's the final step before makeup—or no makeup. (Believe it or not, I do leave the house sometimes with no makeup on!)

Now, if you don't have the patience for a multistep skin care routine, you can look for a moisturizer packed with extras, like SPF, antiaging ingredients, and/or antioxidants. You'll get some of the benefits without all the steps.

DO I NEED NECK CREAM?

I don't use neck cream. Because I apply my sunscreen, retinoid cream, serum, and moisturizer to my neck and chest, I feel that I'm doing enough for that part of my body. But when applying your facial products, don't neglect that area. A lot of people devote all their time to their faces, forgetting that the area right below their jawline needs love too!

DON'T FORGET YOUR HANDS!

It's so easy to neglect your hands and take them for granted. I already mentioned that your hands need sunscreen, but they need moisturizer too. Get in the habit of carrying around a small hand cream in your handbag, makeup bag, or school bag. You can buy a sample-size hand cream, or just refill a small container with your body lotion. Whenever I stay at a hotel, I keep the small bottle of body lotion because it's the perfect portable size.

After you wash your hands (and I hope you wash your hands frequently—it's a good-health must!), apply some lotion. Look for a body lotion or hand cream that contains sun protection and your product can do double duty.

Feet First!

Since we're talking about body parts, let's talk feet! You definitely need to pay attention to your feet. They really take a beating, especially because women's shoes are not very forgiving. And nothing is nastier than neglected feet. You know what I'm talking about—dry, gross, crusty skin. Icky. It happens to me when I wear open-toed shoes a lot. To combat this, I grab a tub of Vaseline, slather it on my feet, and throw on some socks. Any socks will do. Wear them to bed and the next morning, your feet are baby-butt soft. I swear!

FIGHTING ACNE

As I mentioned earlier, acne is a disease. Some people get mild acne, meaning a pimple here and there. Others suffer from painful cysts that form underneath the skin. If your acne is bad, you should see a dermatologist. Many insurance companies cover dermatologist visits and acne medicine. Don't suffer needlessly. Go get help.

You can definitely do things on your own to help your skin too. Some of them we've discussed already, such as removing your makeup and cleansing your skin daily.

You can also use special products designed for acne-prone skin. You will find that almost all of these products contain an ingredient called benzoyl peroxide, which helps clear pores and fight bacteria. Just be careful not to overdo it. You don't want to strip your skin and dry it out. Instead of helping your acne, you'll wind up with acne plus angry, red, irritated skin.

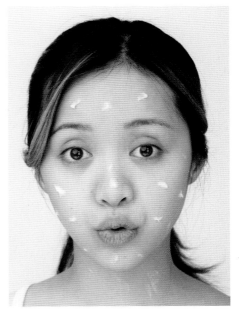

Don't be afraid to moisturize. Just use a lightweight product. Be careful when exfoliating your skin. Avoid any kind of manual scrub or microdermabrasion product. It will exacerbate your problem. If you want to use a chemical exfoliant, check with your dermatologist first.

Another overlooked treatment option is diet. I'm not talking about the old fallacy that chocolate and fried foods cause acne. Some people eat junk food all the time and have nice, clear skin. Life is unfair that way. But all of our bodies are different, including the way our skin reacts to food. Maybe certain foods, like those with dairy or wheat, are exacerbating your skin care issues. You can get tested for food allergies. If your diet isn't that healthy, take steps to improve it. Eat more fresh fruits and vegetables, swap soda for water and green tea, and cut down on processed food. Acne or no acne, you'll feel better eating healthier, and you never know. It could help your complexion.

HOW TO EXFOLIATE

Exfoliating is nothing more than removing the top layer of dead skin cells. It's a great way to brighten and perk up your complexion. As I mentioned earlier, there are a variety of ways to exfoliate. You can use a manual scrub, which is a product that contains a granular element you literally rub on your face (gently, please!) to remove the dead skin cells. Chemical and fruit peels, on the other hand, do the work for you. You just apply and they eat away at the top layer. Be careful with these. They can cause irritation and aren't for everyone. You don't need to exfoliate daily. Try doing it once a week and see how that works for you. My favorite way to exfoliate is with a skin brush. I love the Clarisonic brushes, which are battery operated and use sonic technology to polish and deeply cleanse your skin. It doesn't spin, although it feels like it does when you hold it against your skin. Instead, it oscillates.

EXFOLIATE YOUR LIPS

Do your lips get dry easily? Mine do, so I try to exfoliate them on a regular basis to remove any dead skin. Nothing looks worse than lipstick applied over yucky, flaky skin. So here's a yummy DIY way to exfoliate your lips. Mix a teaspoon of honey with a teaspoon of sugar or salt and gently scrub the mixture on your lips with your fingers, an old toothbrush, a mascara wand, or a spoolie brush. (Obviously, make sure the brush is clean before you use it!) Remove the mixture with a warm washcloth. Apply some balm and you're good to go.

If you do have flaky lips, don't ever pull at the dry bits. You might wind up pulling off too much and you'll start bleeding. That will look even worse than what you started with.

BODY BASICS

What about the skin on the rest of your body? Well, that needs love too. It's not just about your face, after all. I apply body lotion daily and you might want to as well, especially if you have dry skin. I also scrub in the shower using exfoliating gloves.

KP DUTY

Do you ever get those red, ugly bumps on your upper arms (and sometimes your legs)? It's a condition known as keratosis pilaris, or KP, and it's easy to treat. You can't scrub them away, although a lot of people try to do that. You'll need a glycolic acid lotion to make them disappear. You can buy these lotions over the counter, but you should talk to your dermatologist before using them to make sure they're right for you.

CLEAN LIVING

I'm sure you know this, but eating well and exercising are great for your skin. Let's start with diet. The Mayo Clinic, which is a famous organization in the United States focused on medical care, research, and education, has a list of skin-friendly foods. They are:

- Carrots, apricots, and other yellow and orange fruits and vegetables
- Spinach and other green leafy vegetables
- Tomatoes
- Blueberries
- Beans, peas, and lentils
- Salmon, mackerel, and other fatty fish
- Nuts

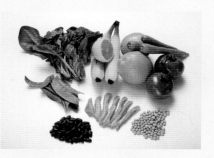

Try incorporating these foods into your diet. If you eat junk food, try to eat less or none at all. Swap sugary soft drinks for water or green tea, as I mentioned. If you can't let go of soda because you love your bubbles, try sparkling water. And plan your meals ahead of time so there's more opportunity to eat food that's fresh and healthy, rather than processed.

As for exercise, get moving! Find an activity that allows you to break a sweat, increase your heart rate, and get your circulation going. You'll flush toxins from your body and benefit your complexion immensely.

DON'T SMOKE!

Smoking is one of the worst things you can do to your skin, and your health in general. Smoking contributes to wrinkles and can result in a sallow complexion. Don't smoke if you want nice skin. It's that simple. If you don't smoke but are considering it, try to resist. Once you start, it's very hard to stop.

GET GLOWING

There's a reason why people think I look like a teenager when I'm not wearing makeup. It's because of my skin care secrets, which aren't secrets anymore! Good luck figuring out your skin care routine; I hope the information I've shared is helpful to you. It's a nice feeling waking up in the morning to good skin, and I wish that for all of you.

Now we're ready to talk about makeup.

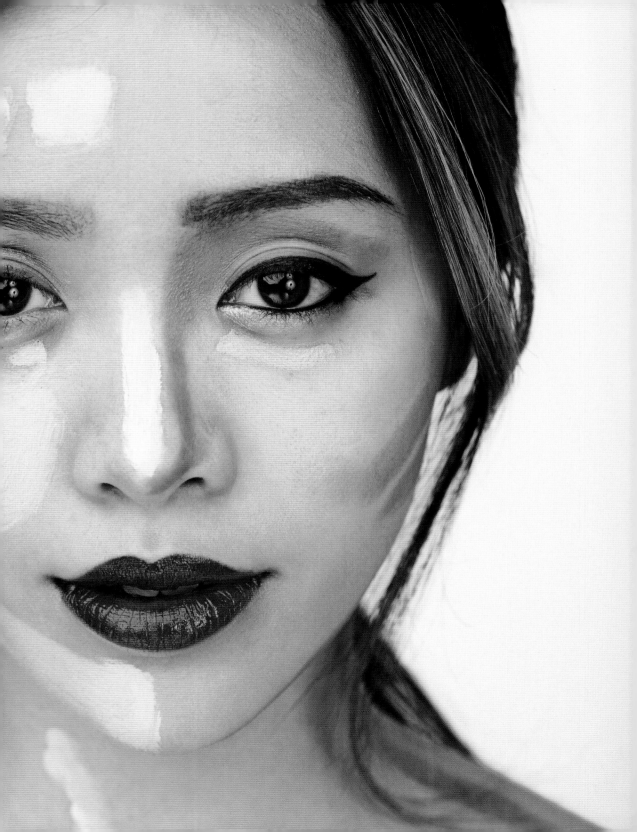

MAKEUP BASICS AND BEYOND

don't need to tell you how much I love makeup. If you know anything about me, you know it's a huge part of my life. First and foremost, it represents my livelihood. Yes, a lot of the credit for my success goes to technology and social media, especially YouTube—but without makeup, would any of this have been possible? Do you think I would have found the same audience if I had made cooking tutorials? Imagine it: "Okay, time to make fried chicken!" Or workout videos? "Fifteen reps, people! C'mon!"

Who knows? What I do know is that makeup has become the way I express my artistry, my creativity, and my desire to share knowledge with others. But I don't want to get all super serious about makeup because it's something that should be fun. I'm always bummed when I meet someone and she tells me she's intimidated by makeup. There's no need for that! If you make a mistake or you don't like what you've just applied, you wash it off and start over. Don't you wish everything in life were like that?

Also, makeup is our war paint! Don't you feel ready to take on the world when you apply your makeup, even when it's just a swipe of lipstick?

Applying makeup is therapeutic. You're taking time for yourself and putting your best face forward. You're being creative and tapping into the artist who dwells inside you. It's great for your psyche. Sure, applying makeup can be a pain when you're in a rush and trying to run out the door to get to work or school on time. Or maybe you don't feel that confident about choosing or applying makeup. I'm going to help you with that. Once you master makeup, you'll feel better and enjoy the process more. And the sharper your application skills, the faster you can get out of the house in the morning!

In this chapter, we're going to talk about a variety of makeup topics. We'll cover some basics, because maybe you're a newbie to the world of makeup, or perhaps you could benefit from a refresher course. We'll also cover some advanced practices. Why not? It's fun to push our skills and see what we're capable of.

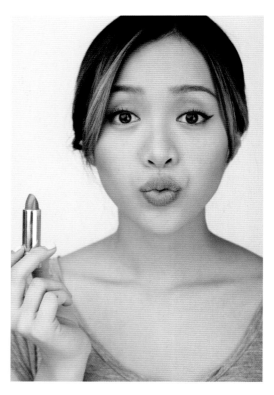

MY MOOD, MY MAKEUP

Who do you want to be today? That's another beautiful thing about makeup. You can wake up one person and leave the house someone else, and it's perfectly acceptable! I often base my look on my mood. If I want to appear more confident, I'll rock some dark lipstick, or maybe a strong eye paired with dramatic brows. If I'm feeling quiet and contemplative, my makeup reflects that. Sometimes I don't wear any makeup at all. Whatever I choose, my whole demeanor changes.

For me, makeup is about telling your story; it's celebrating the different moments in your life with a few subtle changes of liner, lipstick, and shadow.

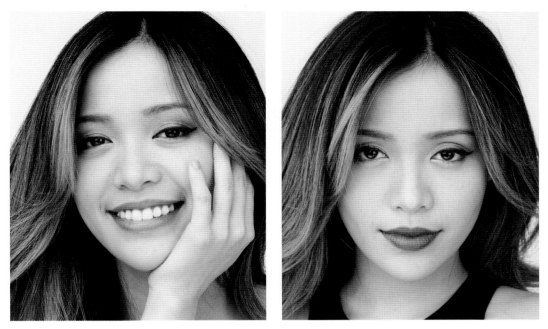

A woman's life is so multifaceted. Do you act the same with your significant other as you do with your mom or dad or as you do with your friends or coworkers? Probably not. Nobody is the same person 100 percent of the time. Nobody has to be! That's why I love being a woman. We can change our looks because makeup gives us that option. Wearing or not wearing makeup represents the freedom to express how we feel and to be who we want to be.

YOUR TOOL KIT

The best place to start talking about makeup is with the tools you need. Just like a carpenter is useless without a hammer or a hairstylist needs scissors, you need the right tools to apply your makeup well. This doesn't mean you need to go out and spend a fortune on makeup brushes and various implements. After all, the best tool is right in front of you: You can apply eye shadow, foundation, concealer, cream blush, lipstick, and contouring and highlighting products so easily with your fingers. (You might not believe this, but you can even do a smoky eye with your fingers.) But your fingers don't work for everything—powder blush, for example. And face powder is pretty tricky to apply with your fingers!

smoky eye—finger-paint style

The index finger provides the most control, so use it to contour.

The middle finger is for the darkest color.

Your ring finger is the most delicate finger, so use it to blend.

Use your pinky finger for the lightest shade, which will be your highlighter.

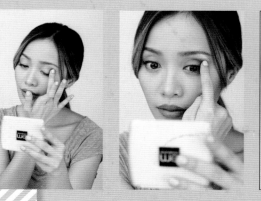

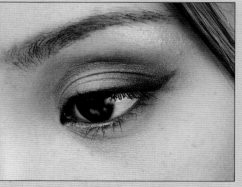

Nice makeup brushes are always a good investment because they can last for years, if not decades. It's true! You just need to take care of them. That means storing them properly and not tossing them mindlessly in the bottom of your purse or crowding them into your makeup bag. You also need to wash them on a regular basis, which we'll discuss shortly.

What do you look for in a good brush? You want a substantial handle that feels good when you hold it, and there should be a generous number of bristles. Run the bristles over the back of your hand and make sure they feel soft and secure. If a few hairs fall out, that's okay. But a brush that loses hairs every time you use it? That's not okay. Return it and ask for a refund.

Also, you have two choices when it comes to bristles: natural hair or synthetic hair. Both are great options and perform equally well. Vegans and vegetarians prefer the synthetic brushes. If that is your preference, make sure to ask what the bristles are made of before you purchase.

If you can't afford an entire collection of nice brushes, start small with a powder brush, a blush brush, and—maybe my favorite—a foundation brush with synthetic bristles. I use mine every time I apply makeup. These three essentials are good investments, and you'll be happy to have them.

A FEW EXTRAS

I know several makeup artists who love applying foundation with a makeup sponge. These come in all sizes and shapes and range in price from cheap to expensive. (Some of the inexpensive drugstore sponges are great, so don't feel you need to spend a fortune.) What you choose depends on your personal preference. You can use the sponge either dry or damp. Some artists think a damp sponge results in a nicer, smoother foundation application, but I find both ways work equally well.

Powder puffs can be used for powdering your face and blending your blush. Most pressed powders come with a puff, but they're not always the best quality. However, they're fine for little touch-ups throughout the day.

Last, always have a few cotton swabs on hand. These are essential for cleaning up tiny mistakes or perfecting lip liner or eyeliner application. When correcting any errors, use the swab dry, or dip it in some eye makeup remover.

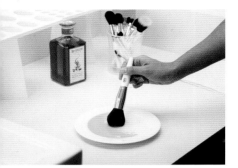

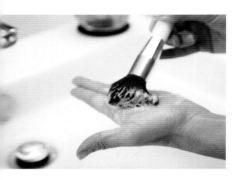

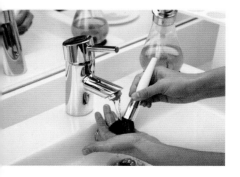

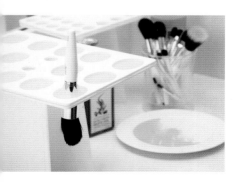

DIRTY BRUSHES? YUCK!

When is the last time you cleaned your makeup brushes? I hope the answer isn't "never"! You definitely need to wash your brushes on a regular basis. I get lazy about this and I'm sure some of you do too, but it's a practice we all need to make a habit, just like brushing our teeth and taking off our makeup each night. Why? Two reasons. First, dirt, oil, and product accumulate on our brushes. Every time we use them, we're redepositing the buildup on our skin, and that's not a good thing, especially for those of us prone to breakouts. Second, you will always get a better result working with clean tools. Every painter knows that to be true.

You should give your brushes what I call a spa treatment once every two weeks, and more frequently if possible. You don't need to spend a lot of money on fancy brush cleaner. All you need is extra-virgin olive oil and antibacterial dishwashing soap. The oil is for reconditioning the bristles and the soap is for getting them clean. Just put the oil and soap on a plate and swirl your dry brush through the two ingredients. You will see the product and pigment coming right off the brush and into the soap-oil mixture. Next, wipe the brush back and forth on the palm of your hand to remove more of the product and pigment. Then run lukewarm water over the brush until the water runs clear. Your brushes will look and feel brand-spanking new.

I actually learned this trick in an art class when we needed to clean oil paints from our brushes. If you've worked with this kind of paint, you know how difficult it can be to remove. The reason people have loved oil paintings over the years is because the colors last the longest compared to all other paints. So you can imagine what happens when oil paint is on your paintbrush! It's essential to clean those brushes daily.

To dry your makeup brushes, blot them with a paper

towel to remove any excess water. Dry them upside down if you can, so that water doesn't seep into the barrel. The bristles are held in place with glue and you don't want to loosen up the glue. Also, water can cause warping and rusting, and you don't want to change the integrity of the brush. If upside down isn't an option, you can dry them sideways. Just put the brushes on a towel and let them air-dry. Never use a hair dryer or put the brushes on a radiator or heated surface.

Synthetic bristles tend to dry quickly, but natural bristles take longer. A large powder brush can take a full day to dry; smaller brushes will take less time. Keep that in mind and plan accordingly. You don't want to discover that all of your brushes are wet when you need to do your makeup in a rush or for an important occasion!

If you use sponges and puffs, don't forget to wash them on a regular basis too. A foaming face wash or gentle baby shampoo is the best option. Dishwashing detergent is too harsh for these items.

> TIP: Are your brushes looking and feeling a little grimy, but you don't have time for a proper cleaning? To quickly refresh them, use baby wipes to wipe down the bristles.

MY EVERYDAY ROUTINE

Before we get into the details of each part of the face, I thought I'd talk about my daily makeup routine. I apply my makeup in a specific order, and I'll explain why. Then we'll talk more about individual products and application techniques.

Brows—I do this before eyes, lips, and cheeks because brows are the frame for the face.

Primer—This provides a base for my makeup and keeps it bulletproof all day long.

Foundation—This evens out my skin tone.

Concealer—This covers any dark areas (such as under-eye circles) or redness that my foundation doesn't.

Powder—This sets everything, reduces shine, and helps my makeup last.

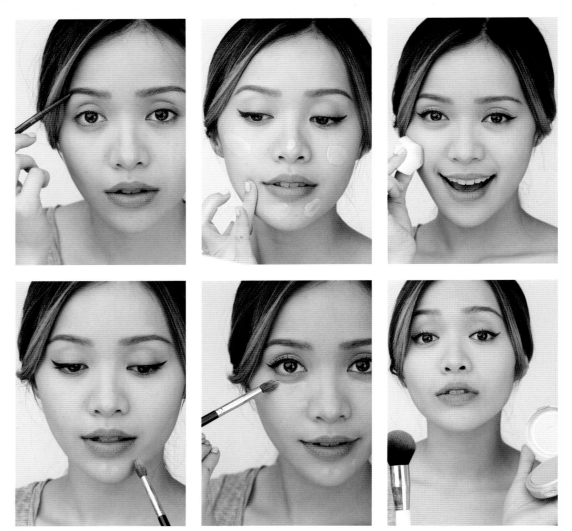

Your everyday look should look as if you had 10 hours of sleep. Thankfully we have makeup here to help us.

Next, I do whatever part of my face I'm emphasizing that day. If I'm doing a smoky eye, I'll do my eyes first. If I'm doing a beautifully lined dark lip, I'll do that first. This way everything is in proportion. You want to make sure to balance your look. That means making one thing the focal point on your face and toning down everything else. For example, if you do a major eye look, keep the lips and cheeks neutral. Bright red lips? Be subtle with your eyes and cheeks. It's all about the ratio. You don't want to overwhelm your face. When someone looks at you, his or her first thought should never be, "Whoa. That's a lot of makeup."

The very last thing I do is apply mascara. It's the final touch, like setting your hair with hairspray.

FACE FIRST

Let's talk about face makeup. This category covers everything you need to prime and perfect your complexion. You want a nice, smooth canvas before you apply the rest of your makeup, and these products help you achieve that.

PRIMER

Are you familiar with this product? Primer does exactly what it says. It primes your face and helps your makeup adhere better. Have you ever painted a room? Usually, you put a layer of primer on the walls before you apply any color. It's the same principle. Look for a product identified as face primer, makeup primer, or foundation primer. They all do the same thing. However, some include ingredients that mattify, control oil, fight acne, boost radiance, etc. Pick what's best for your skin.

Apply a thin layer of primer with your fingers or a clean foundation brush to moisturized skin. Let it dry for at least ten seconds. If you're applying primer to your entire face, you really don't need more than a quarter-size amount. If you're applying to your T-zone only, you need even less. My T-zone gets oily, so I always need extra help in that area to keep my makeup in place. If I need my makeup to be impeccable and long lasting on a particular day, I apply primer to my entire face.

Before you run out and buy primer, ask yourself if you really need it. Not everyone does! Does your makeup go on just fine and last for hours without any primer? Then you probably can do without. If your makeup disappears an hour after you apply it, because of the humidity outside or your skin type or another factor, it could be ideal for you. Same if you just want a smoother makeup application. You should never feel compelled to use a product just because it exists or because someone else uses it. Use what you need and what you enjoy wearing.

I wear foundation over my primer, but some women choose to wear primer alone (or maybe topped with a little powder). That might be an option for you if your skin tone is even and you just need a little boost.

FOUNDATION

This is a product used to even out your skin tone. Unlike primer, which is generally colorless, foundation is pigmented. The idea is that you choose a foundation similar to your skin tone and it helps give your complexion a nice, smooth, uniform look. If you don't have great skin—and who has great skin every day of the year?—foundation can help you fake it.

Choosing a foundation can be confusing because there are thousands of options on the market. Hopefully the information I'm about to share will simplify the process for you. You should sample a variety of foundation formulas to see what's right for you and your skin type. Foundation is one of the more expensive makeup products out there, so don't waste your money buying the wrong one.

TYPES OF FOUNDATION

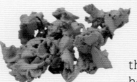

Liquid foundation—This is the most popular. It comes in a bottle (or sometimes a tube) and ranges from thin to thick in consistency. The thinner the formula, the lighter the coverage. The thicker, the heavier.

Tinted moisturizer—This is exactly what it sounds like, moisturizer that's been tinted to provide some coverage. You can use it in place of moisturizer, or use it over moisturizer for an extra layer of hydration. You'll find that tinted moisturizer is thicker than most moisturizers.

Cream foundation—This comes in a compact or stick form and is soft and sometimes even bouncy in texture. It is not liquidy at all.

Mineral foundation—This is a colored powder made of minerals. The recommended application technique is buffing the powder onto your skin with a special brush.

Powder foundation or foundation powder—This is a form of pressed powder that provides color and coverage.

Airbrush foundation—This comes in a can or spray mechanism that releases a fine mist of foundation. Coverage can be on the heavy side. There are airbrush machines that you can buy, but they tend to be very expensive and are mostly used by movie and theatrical makeup artists.

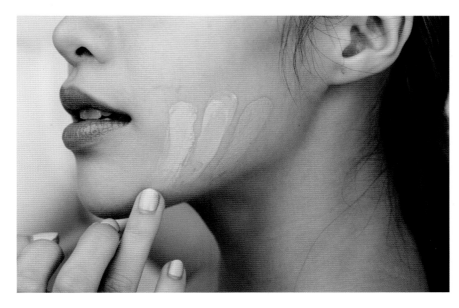

Which color
disappears on
your skin?

How to Select the Perfect Foundation

Don't test potential foundations on the back of your hand or on your inner arm. If you're at a store that lets you try on product, pick the three shades closest to your complexion color. (Beware of foundations that skew too yellow, pink, or red.) Take each one and paint a sheer stripe on the area between your cheek and jawline. Walk outside into daylight and see how it looks. If you're at the mall, browse around for twenty minutes. Some foundation formulas can oxidize and change color, so you need to let a little time pass to see if that happens. What you want is a color that blends seamlessly into your skin. If these colors don't work, keep looking. You will find the foundation that's perfect for you. You just need to do some leg-work.

It's not that different from finding the perfect mate. You have to spend time with a few before you commit to one!

Skin Tone Versus Undertone

Understanding your skin tone and your undertone can help you find the right foundation. Your skin tone is the color of your skin. That can change over time or throughout the year, depending on how much sun you get. Your undertone, however, never changes. It's literally a tone—either cool, warm, or neutral—that radiates from beneath your skin. Choose a foundation that matches your skin tone but that skews in the direction of your undertone. So let's say you need a beige foundation. If your undertone is warm, pick a beige that feels warmer. Maybe it has a bit of yellow to it or is just a bit brighter. If you're cool toned, look for a beige that feels a bit more icy or cool.

If you can't tell just by looking at your skin, there are a few other ways to figure out your undertone. What clothing colors do you wear the most? You probably gravitate toward the colors that are most flattering for you. Do you like warmer colors or cooler colors? Some examples of warm colors are pumpkin, camel, peach, brown, and olive. Think colors associated with autumn. Some cool colors are sky blue, navy, white, violet, lavender, gray, and pink. How about jewelry? Do you look best in gold (warm) or silver (cool)?

Last, look at your veins. Blue veins signal a cool undertone. Green, warm. And if you're somewhere in between, you could have a neutral undertone.

Mix Master

Even though there are countless foundation and concealer shades on the market, there's still a chance you might not find the perfect shade for you at a beauty counter. In that case, it's fine to mix two colors to get the right one. Professional makeup artists do this all the time. It's just like an artist painting a picture. You've seen an artist's palette, with bits of color all over it, right? The painter dabs his or her brush into the various colors and combines them to get the perfect shade.

The Right Foundation Type

Shade isn't the only consideration when it comes to foundation. You need to think about your skin type and texture as well. Whatever your skin care concern, there's a foundation for you. If you have oily skin, for example, you don't want a hydrating foundation formula. You want something water based and mattifying. Do you need to fight acne? Want some antiaging help? Options exist for all of that.

You might need to rotate among two or three different foundations

What is BB cream?

BB creams first appeared in Korea and were so popular that dozens of beauty brands launched their own versions. Basically, BB creams are tinted moisturizers that come loaded with extras—SPF, antioxidants, treatment ingredients, primer, etc. The BB stands for "beauty balm" or "blemish balm." I love using BB creams, but it's unclear if they are a fad or will have staying power. Now you've even got CC creams, which stands for "color correcting" or "color control." I wonder how long until we get through the rest of the alphabet! If you're curious about BB cream, ask for a sample next time you're near a beauty counter that sells it.

throughout the year. Sometimes a single foundation doesn't fit all of your needs. If the climate where you live changes dramatically—hot and humid one day, cold and dry the next—you might want to switch it up based on the weather report. Or perhaps it's your skin color that changes. Maybe you're tan certain times of the year. You'll need a lighter shade and a darker one to mix and match with your complexion.

Coverage

You know your skin tone and undertone and you've considered the skin care benefits you want in your foundation. Next, you need to decide what kind of coverage you want. What does that mean exactly? Do you like or need heavier makeup? Maybe you rock a really retro made-up look. Or perhaps you have some acne scarring you would like to cover up. Look for words like *matte, velvet,* and *full coverage* in the name of the foundation. Want just a light veil of coverage? Look for words like *Sheer, lightweight,* and *natural.*

Application tools

You have a number of options for applying foundation. As I mentioned, I love foundation brushes. These are medium-size brushes with synthetic bristles that are flat, rather than puffy or curved like a powder brush. They provide a lot of control and help you apply that perfect thin layer of foundation every time. Other application options are your fingers or a sponge. As I mentioned earlier, some makeup artists prefer to use a damp sponge for foundation because they feel it results in a smoother finish. Try it yourself and see what you prefer.

Does everyone need foundation?

Not at all! If you have an even skin tone, you might choose to skip foundation and use concealer and/or powder. It depends on what's right for you.

Where do I use foundation?

It depends on how much coverage you want. You can use it over your entire face, but you will look more "made up." I prefer to use foundation where I need it, so I spot-treat. That means I apply it to the places where I have redness or where I need to even out my skin tone, such as around my nose and on my cheeks. I like to start with a thin layer of foundation, then add another layer if needed. Most foundations are buildable, meaning you can apply layer upon layer. Just don't overdo it. If you apply too much, especially all at once, it can look cakey.

Don't forget your neck when applying foundation. You don't need to cover your entire neck, but be sure to smooth the foundation over your jawline and down toward your neck. You don't want an obvious line separating your face and your neck. If they are completely different colors, you can extend your foundation down your neck and chest so everything looks even hued. Just be sure to pick a transfer-resistant foundation that won't get on your clothing.

CONCEALER

This is a heavily pigmented cream designed to conceal spots, redness, and dark circles. It differs from foundation in terms of texture and coverage level.

Pimple Coverage

You want to think like a painter when covering pimples. I use a concealer brush and apply thin layers of concealer right over the pimple. Don't slop on too much concealer all at

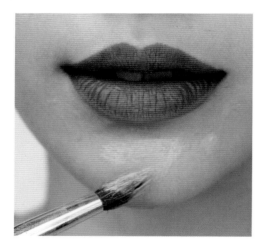

once. The pimple will look cakey and/or bumpy. With a very light hand, build light layer upon layer until the pimple disappears. Using the brush, blur the edges of the concealer into the skin around the pimple so everything blends and looks natural. Then, ever so gently, put some powder over the concealer to set it. Do not touch the area until you need a touch-up. Keep your hair, fingers, and phone away from the spot! Nothing can ruin makeup like pressing your phone against your face. Check your makeup at midday to make sure everything still looks good.

How do I use concealer?
You can use it over foundation for those areas that need extra help, such as acne scars, pimples, and/or under-eye circles. Or you can use it alone, on top of bare skin, if you just need spot coverage.

Concealer Cue

Concealer should be one or two shades lighter than your skin tone. When you're concealing, you're generally trying to cover something darker, so you want product that is lighter.

Cover Dark Circles

You never want your concealer to be so light that you look like a reverse raccoon. Yes, your concealer should be lighter, but not dramatically so. If you have dark circles, you want a thicker concealer that will provide ample coverage. Otherwise, it won't have enough oomph to cover anything. You can use your fingers to apply, but I find a concealer brush gives more control. Put a bit of product on the back of your hand and dab the brush into it lightly. You want to build the concealer in layers; you don't want to glob all the product on at once. Work around your tear duct (which is at the inside corner of your eye) and under the eye, covering wherever you have darkness. Apply a second and third layer as necessary, working in very thin layers. Some people have redness right under their lash line, which makes them look tired, so you can apply a thin layer of concealer there as well.

Next, you need to decide whether to powder under your eyes or not. This part of the face is very delicate and can be dry too. However, concealer under your eyes can move around and bunch up, rather than stay smooth. If that happens to you, powder can keep everything in place. There are special setting powders designed for under the eyes, but I use pressed powder and it works just fine. Apply with a light hand and a small brush or puff.

Can I use my foundation as concealer?
Absolutely. If your foundation provides the coverage you need, go ahead and use it to cover spots and to brighten your under-eye area. If you need more help covering acne scars or dark circles, go with concealer, because it has more ability to, well, conceal, just as its name says.

Don't Hide Your Tattoo!
Yes, you can use concealer to hide your tattoo, but why would you? It's a piece of art that represents your story. In the past, girls with tattoos were considered wild, but that's an old-fashioned way of thinking. Today, tattoos are about self-expression. Let the world see yours and celebrate it!

POWDER

You know what powder is, but what does it do for your face? If you are wearing foundation and concealer, powder will set your makeup. Foundation and concealer tend to be creamy products that can slip and slide around, so powder keeps them in place and helps your makeup last throughout the day. If you have oily skin, powder also keeps shine under control.

TYPES OF POWDER

Pressed powder—This is solid powder that comes in a compact.

Loose powder—This is ground down to a light and fluffy texture.

Translucent powder—This is a sheer, colorless powder that can be used on all skin tones. However, I've seen colored powders labeled as translucent, so be careful what you buy.

Setting powder—All powders set your makeup, but some are marked specifically as setting powders. These tend to be loose or pressed powders that are truly translucent and compatible with many skin tones.

Foundation powder—A heavier pressed powder that provides coverage similar to that of a liquid foundation.

Mineral powder—A type of powder, loose or pressed, made of minerals.

BROW KNOW-HOW

Brows don't inspire love letters and poetry the same way eyes and lips can, but they are so important to a beautifully made-up face. You might not realize it, but brows frame your look and give it structure.

SYMMETRY/ASYMMETRY

Your brows don't need to look identical. Most people have naturally asymmetric faces, so you might find one of your brows is higher than the other or shaped differently. As long as they look similar, you don't need to stress over making them look exactly alike. I always like to say, brows are sisters, not twins.

If you're going to tweeze them yourself, look at your brows and see what their natural shape is. Don't go in and randomly tweeze hairs. I want you to have a plan. Decide what shape you want. I advise looking through fashion and beauty magazines and finding pictures of celebrities and models whose brows you like. Look for an eye shape and face shape similar to

How do I tweeze my brows?

I'm so glad you asked. If you're going to tweeze your brows yourself, undertweeze rather than overtweeze. This is so important! Fuller brows always look more youthful and fresh than thin brows, despite what might be in style at the moment. The danger of overtweezing is that the hair may not grow back. Don't believe me? A lot of women (and some men) have learned this lesson the hard way.

   If you are new to tweezing, it's best to go to an expert and have your brows done professionally. The brow expert will shape them and give you a nice framework to follow. (Get recommendations first! Do not go to a brow expert if you've never seen his or her work in person. Pictures don't count.)

yours. Plenty of celebs have awesome brows, but that doesn't mean their brows will work on your face.

Next, you're going to take a white eyeliner pencil and draw right over the hairs you don't want. This is your guide for where to tweeze. With a good sharp pair of tweezers, pluck one hair at a time. Never pull out a clump of hair! That's painful and won't provide the precision we're looking for.

If the area you are tweezing hurts, put an ice cube in a paper towel and hold it over your skin. That should take away some of the pain.

Brow pencil or brow powder?
For softer, feathery brows, I like powder. If you want more sharpness and precision, traditional pencil is the way to go. I actually use a combination of the two: powder to soften my brows, then the pencil to make tiny strokes and create the illusion of little hairs. As for the color you choose, it depends on your brow and hair color. If you have darker hair, go lighter. Light hair, go darker, but just a bit. If you want a high-fashion look, go with really dark brows.

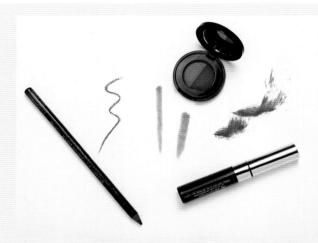

MEET THE SPOOLIE

The name is silly, but I love my spoolie! It looks like a miniature version of the brush you use to clean the inside of bottles. A spoolie is essential for nicely groomed brows. You can use it to brush your brows and blend your brow makeup into place. It softens any harsh edges. If you overpenciled, brush the spoolie over the area and you'll see the color blend in. Some eyebrow pencils have built-in spoolies. (You also can use it to unclump any clumpy mascara, and if you have a clean spoolie, you can use it to exfoliate your lips.)

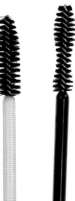

EYE SPY

Nothing can change your look the way eye makeup can. Think about the difference between dramatic smoky eyes with big full lashes, and demure liquid liner. It's major, right? But nothing befuddles women like eye makeup. It's the hardest makeup to master. The best eye makeup advice I have? Lock yourself in your bathroom and start playing. No one has to see your experiments until you decide which looks you love! Practice does make perfect in this case.

KNOW YOUR EYES

People have different eyelid and eye shapes, so it's important to know yours in order to bring out the best in your features. Look in the mirror and gaze into your eyes. It might feel silly, but go for it. Now, with your eyes open, look at your eyelids. How much eyelid real estate, as I like to call it, do you

have? Are your lids barely visible, or do you have a lot of space there? Flip through some beauty and fashion magazines to find models and actresses with eyes similar to yours. Look at their makeup and try to copy it. You don't need to leave the house in that makeup, but you'll learn a lot about your eye shape and what works for you.

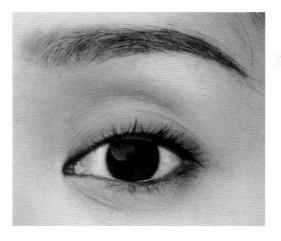

Don't get frustrated by what you can't do. Just because you don't have a large lid space doesn't mean you can't have fun with different eye makeup looks. It's all about honing your techniques. I've seen women with different lid shapes and sizes rock all eye makeup looks. Don't box yourself in! Play and experiment.

EYE MAKEUP PRIMER

One of my favorite products is eyelid primer, which is a base that goes on under your eye shadow. It helps prevent fading and creasing, and if you have oily eyelids, it's especially useful. If you want your eye shadow to last all day, prime away! Eye primer also will help intensify the color payoff of your eye shadows. You'll see the difference right away. Some eye primers have a creamy texture; others have a more silicone feel, which allows the eye shadow to glide right on. I recommend trying on as many primers as you can to find the one that suits your eyes best.

I don't recommend primer under your eyes, however. That area is very delicate and you don't want too many products there. Things can start to look cakey if you layer on too much.

When you're ready to start your eye makeup, the primer should be the first thing you apply. Just use your fingers to dab it on, then blend it out from your lids, over your crease, and up to your brow bone. Wherever you want to add color, add the primer there first! Then wait for it to dry (I say thirty seconds) and your eyes will be primed and ready to go.

NEUTRAL EYE SHADOW

No matter what stage of eye makeup expertise you're at, you can never go wrong with neutrals. These are any matte or slightly shimmery colors in earth tones or flesh tones. Think creams, nudes, tans, browns, and grays. Neutrals are hard to mess up. You can wear a single color, or use multiple colors for a smoky or contoured eye. Always work from light to dark, because you can layer and build up the color without needing to remove any product.

RAINBOW COLORS

Perhaps you're not a neutral kind of person. You're the person who loves the big box of crayons. Go ahead and have fun with color! If you feel bold or know what colors work for you, by all means use them. You'll always look great when you're being yourself.

That is, except for red eye shadow! Red eye shadow will make your eyes appear tired and irritated. Most people should avoid using red. However, don't let me steer you away from this passionate color if you love it! In Japan, geisha still use red makeup around their eyes to make them look more alluring. It just goes to show, there are no wrong colors. It's all about how you wear them.

EYELINER

There are so many types of eyeliner and so many ways to apply them! Pencil, pot, liquid, powder. Feeling sexy? Try lining along the top and bottom waterline. Innocent? Lightly line the top eyelid. Punky? Smudge that liner around your entire eye. Fashion-forward? Wing your eyeliner out to the sides. You have lots of options.

PENCIL EYELINER

I like to think of pencil eyeliner as the most basic eye makeup you can start with. It's the most forgiving and easy to use. If you can write with a pencil, you can draw with an eyeliner pencil. After all, what you're doing is essentially writing/drawing on your lids.

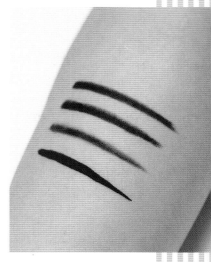

There are two varieties of pencils: 1) Mechanical, which you twist upward when you need more product. You don't need a sharpener for this one. 2) Traditional, which you need to sharpen. This is my favorite kind of pencil because you can get a much finer point than with a mechanical pencil. It lets you be more precise and gives you control over the type of look you want.

> TIP: *Don't make your pencil too sharp! There's no danger of hurting yourself, but the point can snap off and you'll waste precious time and product.*

EYE SHADOW AS EYELINER

Did you know you can use any eye shadow as liner? It's super easy. All you need is the shadow and a liner brush. If you want a sharp, precise line, wet the brush. You can use water, but I prefer eye drops, which adhere better to the powder than water does. A dry brush plus powder creates a beautiful hazy line, which I love because it's more natural looking.

Again, it all depends on the look you're going for!

HOW TO TIGHTLINE YOUR EYES

What does *tightline* even mean? It's a trick that creates the illusion of a nice full-looking lash line and involves lining right along the upper waterline, below the lashes. It's a great no-makeup look—natural with extra oomph. Applying along the upper waterline will take a bit of practice. It's sensitive there and you can easily tear up. Go slow and be gentle. It takes time to get your eyes used to this. Your eyes have a natural reflex, so, of course, you're going to blink like crazy when you're sticking something close to them. Once you've done it for the hundredth time, your eyes will be desensitized and bulletproof like mine. I can now line my eyes in the backseat of a speeding car with no trouble. (However, I do not recommend this!)

LIQUID LINER

If you've never used it, liquid liner is exactly what it sounds like. It comes either in a vial with a thin brush or preloaded into a marker-type applicator. I love liquid liner, but it took me a long time to master! Pencil eyeliners are to writing pencils as liquid liners are to painting or calligraphy! Liquid liners will give you a more fluid line. You can control the line weight better, creating a thin to thick line with just one stroke! It's all about practicing. People find liquid liner the most intimidating of all liners, which is understand-

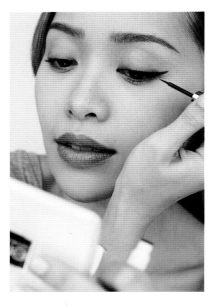

able because it's not as forgiving as pencil. If you mess up, you have to clean it up with eye makeup remover.

Liquid liner is best applied above your upper lash line. You can make the line thick or thin and even wing it out at the ends. I wouldn't use it under your lower lashes or below your eyes, unless you're going for a very theatrical feel or want to look like a high-fashion picture from a magazine.

CREAM EYELINER

This type comes in a little pot and is applied with a brush. It's similar to liquid liner in terms of the looks you can create, except it's more smudgeable and easier to use. Cream also provides different finishes—matte, metallic, or shiny.

MAKE YOUR EYES POP

White or nude eyeliner applied along your lower waterline is a great trick for making your eyes look bigger because it gives the illusion of extending the whites of your eyes. It's also good if you look tired and/or have a lower waterline that is very red. You'll look more refreshed and awake.

Another trick is putting a shimmery shadow or eyeliner around the outside of your tear duct. It's a very fresh, youthful look. Just use your finger to pat it gently in a C-shape around the duct. Don't get it too close to the eye and make sure to blend. You don't want an obvious semicircle of product. As for colors, you can use anything light and shimmery. My personal favorite shade for this trick is rose gold.

HOW TO CURL YOUR LASHES

Do you own a lash curler? To the uninitiated, it's a very intimidating-looking object. For those who know how to use it properly, it's the best

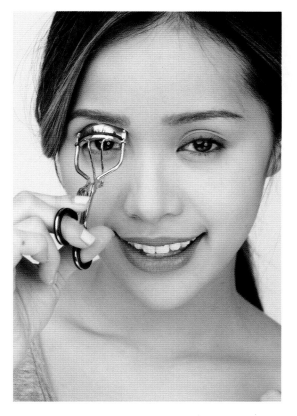

tool for giving your lashes a lift and making your eyes seem more open. Before using your curler, take a look at it. See the curved rubber piece? That serves as a soft base for your lashes. Make sure it's not out of place or worn away. If it is, you could chop off all your lashes. I know only one person to whom this has happened, but I don't want you to be the second!

Open the device and center your lashes between the curved metal top and the rubber base and gently clamp it down. Hold it in place for ten seconds and release. Make sure to get the curler close to the base of your lashes, otherwise you could wind up with a weird crimp in the middle of your lashes. Make sure to curl before you put on your mascara. There's something about the mascara and the metal that makes it easier to pull out your lashes. Bottom line: Be careful!

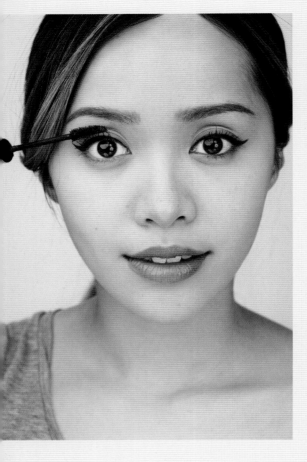

MASCARA

Just like foundation, mascara can be confusing because there are so many choices! There are countless formulas and brush shapes available, and there are always new versions on the market. It's going to take a little trial and error to find the right one for you. Just because a certain mascara works really well on your friend's lashes doesn't mean it will work well on yours. That doesn't make it a bad mascara; it's just that we all have different hair types and that is true of our lashes, too. Some girls have thin hair and thin lashes, some have very thick hair and thick lashes. Know your hair and lash type. I have very thick hair, but my lashes are thin and grow straight down. For that reason, I need a lightweight, drier mascara formula that won't weigh down my lashes even further.

Some women with thin lashes love waterproof mascaras because they tend not to flake, they're long wearing, and the wax-based formulas hold a curl better. I find they make my lashes brittle. As with so many makeup-related matters, it all comes down to what works best for you!

CONDITION YOUR LASHES

As I mentioned earlier, your lashes are no different from the hairs on your head. If you wear a lot of mascara, you should condition your lashes at night. There are various lash treatments you can buy, but plain old petroleum jelly works just fine. That's what I use before I go to bed and my lashes are very conditioned.

Do you need lash primer?

Lash primer is a base coat for your mascara. It helps plump up the lashes by adding an extra layer and gives the mascara something to adhere to. I don't use lash primer because it makes my lashes too heavy. You might find that it works for you if your lashes need some extra oomph.

LIPSTICK, LINER, AND GLOSS

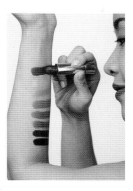

I don't even want to tell you how many lipsticks and glosses I own. Suffice it to say, a lot! But what's more fun and feminine than those two things? Sure, nail polish is a blast, though it does take a bit of skill to apply. Same with eye shadow. But lipstick and lip gloss? They're so easy to play with and apply expertly. Just think how dramatically you can change your look with a quick swipe of lipstick or gloss. A red lipstick speaks volumes—without you saying a single word! A nude color takes you in the absolute opposite direction for a natural look. Tangerine is fun and pinks are fresh, while mauves are sophisticated.

HOW TO LINE YOUR LIPS

Lip liner is such a useful tool, but it can be easily misused. I think we've all seen people who abuse liner and extend their lip lines far, far, far beyond what is appropriate. It doesn't have to be that way! You can create the illusion of fuller-looking lips, but you don't need to totally exaggerate what you have. Think subtle and use a lip pencil that matches your natural lip color. When you're trying to make your lips look bigger, it's best to stick to neutral colors of liner, lipstick, and gloss. Otherwise it can look clownish.

Lip liner also is great if you have an uneven lip shape. Use a lip pencil similar to your natural lip color and even out any irregularity in the outline of your lips. Fill in the rest of your lips if you like. You can wear this alone or top with lipstick and/or gloss. If you've lost pigment in your lips (sometimes that happens to smokers), you can use lip liner to add color back in.

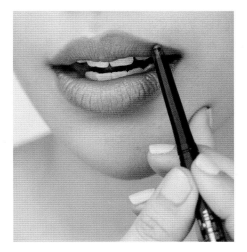

Are you thinking about sporting a red, dark, or bold lip? Lip liner can be the primer for that color. Take a lip liner in a shade that matches your lipstick, and outline your lips. Next, fill in your lips with the pencil. Because liner is drier and less oily than lipstick, it will provide a barrier to prevent your lipstick from feathering and bleeding outside your lip line. (This is a common problem with darker colors.) Once you've colored in your entire lip, apply your lipstick on top.

TIP: If your lips are thin, a bright or bold color will accentuate that. Try using a nude shimmery lip gloss instead. It's great for making your lips look bigger than they are.

DON'T SMOKE!

It's bad enough that we need to deal with pollution in the environment every day. If you smoke or are considering it, you need to know how bad smoking is for your skin, and your lips in particular. It dries out your lips and contributes to lip discoloration. Also, it can cause wrinkles around your lips as you age, and those aren't pretty.

WHAT IS MY CUPID'S BOW?

It's that little V right above the center of your lips. A favorite trick of mine is to highlight the cupid's bow to give the illusion of fuller lips. It's like a 3-D

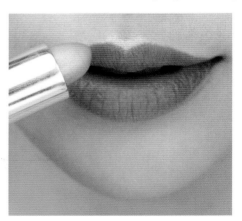

effect. You can use a shimmery white eye shadow and a thin brush, or a white or nude pencil. Just trace along the V after you've applied your liner and/or lipstick and gently blend or soften the V. You don't want to leave the house with a really obvious white V above your lips! Top with gloss and go.

You can give the V a little staying power by priming that area first. Just put a tiny dab of makeup primer or eye shadow primer right in that space and follow the directions as above.

BLUSH BASICS

Whereas lips help you make a statement, blush sets the tone. Of course, you can experiment with different blush looks, but unless you're going to a club, starring in a music video, or living the rock-and-roll life, keep your blush fairly basic. It's fine if people notice your eye shadow or lipstick, but your blush? That's a weird thing for people to comment on. Blush should just complement everything else that's going on.

KNOW YOUR FACE SHAPE

When it comes to blush application, you need to understand your face shape and where blush should be placed for the most flattering effect.

HOW TO FIND YOUR CHEEKBONES

Not sure where your cheekbones are? Just feel your face! Put your fingers on the center of your cheeks and feel for the knobby parts. Those are known as the apples of your cheeks. Now, starting at the apples, feel for the prominent bones that extend all the way toward your ears. Those are your cheekbones.

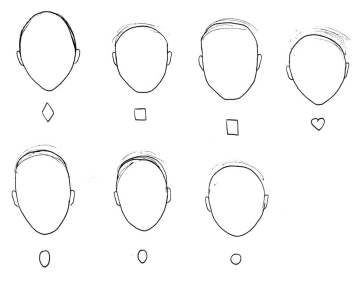

THE BEST BLUSH COLOR

How do you know what's right for you? For me, blush is more about a tone than a color. I'm not a fan of obvious blush colors; I prefer natural shades.

BLEND!

Failure to blend is the number one mistake you can make with blush. Don't leave the house with an identifiable blush "shape" on your face, like a circle or a triangle. Make sure to buff in the color with your brush, a puff, or a sponge. Buffing is just a gentle blending in of the color. But don't be overzealous or you'll wipe off all the product you just applied!

CONTOURING AND HIGHLIGHTING

Contouring and highlighting is a bit of makeup trickery that is beloved by actresses, models, and anyone who has their photo taken frequently. With this, you're playing with light and shadow to emphasize certain parts of your face and de-emphasize others. This is definitely advanced makeup artistry.

Simply put, contouring is about playing with shadows to make certain areas of the face recede so others can pop. Highlighting is about capturing the light to give the illusion of fullness or to spotlight a certain area.

Let's start with contouring. How does it work exactly? Well, first you need to decide on your contouring makeup. You can use any kind of matte powder product—bronzer, eye shadow, pressed powder—or special contouring cream designed just for this purpose. Make sure to pick a neutral color darker than your natural skin tone. I find that bronze or taupe colors work best on me. To apply, you can use a foundation brush or your fingers.

Next, decide what you want to contour. You can make your nose appear smaller and/or thinner by applying contouring makeup along the outside of the bridge of your nose and on the tip of your nose. You can strengthen your jawline by darkening where your actual jawbone is. You can boost your cheekbones by darkening the area underneath the bones and applying blush above the contoured area. Always make sure to blend so you don't walk out of the house with dark stripes on your face.

A little warning about contouring. Not everyone looks good with a contoured face! It can age you and make you look harsh if you do it with a heavy hand. And, truthfully, not everyone needs contour. In Asia they don't contour their cheeks because they want a fuller face, a look they consider more youthful. In the United States, it's the opposite—it's all about cheekbones and a strong, chiseled jawline. Personally, I prefer fullness, which is why I love highlighting. Also, highlighting looks good on everyone.

You can highlight your cheeks, the center of your eyelids, or your brow bone. (The tricks we discussed with highlighting outside your tear duct and along the cupid's bow are examples of highlighting.) Don't highlight your forehead. Highlighting emphasizes an area, so it will only serve to make your forehead look bigger.

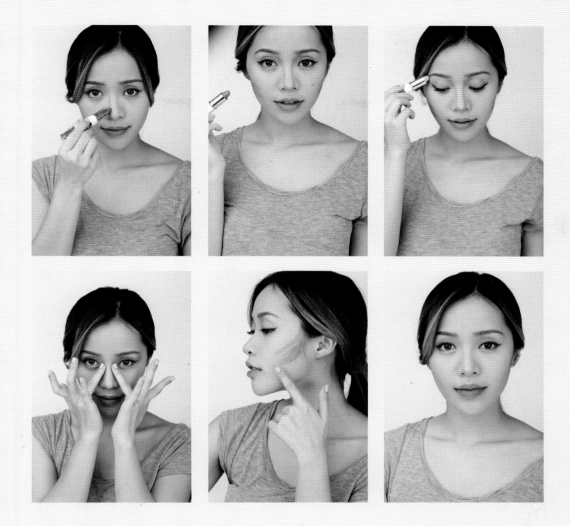

To highlight, you need a nude or off-white shimmery or matte product. You can use either a special highlighting powder or cream, or eye shadow. Again, make sure to blend.

To master contouring and highlighting, give yourself time to study and play. Trial and error is the best way to learn. Sit in front of a mirror and move the lighting around to see where the natural shadows and highlights fall on your face. If you can, dim the light a little and take a picture. Go back in front of the mirror and start re-creating the shadows and highlights, but with a light hand. You want to layer the product a bit at a time. It will look more natural and not as made up.

ORGANIZE YOUR MAKEUP

Keeping your makeup nice and neat is beneficial in so many ways. When you know where everything is, you won't spend precious minutes looking for that item you swear you saw last week. Also, when you're in a rush and everything is disorganized, it's easy to break things. Have you ever been scrambling to get ready and dropped a compact or an eye shadow on the floor? If so, you know what can happen. The product crumbles into bits and becomes unusable. Makeup is fragile, so you need to take care of it. Otherwise you're wasting your time and money.

Before you start organizing, think about your lifestyle and what works best for you. Do you sit in front of a vanity and take your time putting on makeup? Or do you rush into the bathroom with your makeup bag and rush out? I prefer to sit on the floor when I'm putting on makeup. I have a full-length Ikea mirror that leans against the wall, and it's close to a window,

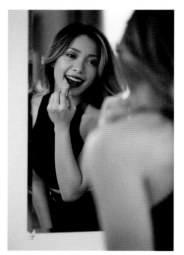

which provides nice light. Natural light is great because it's so unforgiving. You can really see what you're doing!

Also, think about how you like to organize your clothes and accessories. You might have an organization style that comes naturally to you, so you can simply mimic that. Do you organize your clothes by color, by season, or by occasion? Do the same with your makeup.

If organizing doesn't come naturally to you, ask yourself a few other questions. Do you need everything to be practical, portable, and out of sight? Maybe you need a case that you can move from room to room and store in the bottom of your closet. Invest in a makeup case, or buy a tool kit from your local hardware store. These are your tools, after all! Or do you want everything on display in a way that's practical and pretty? Look for beautiful cups and jars and decorative boxes for the top of your dresser. Do you want your room to look like a boutique? Put your products on a magnetic board, so you can grab and go. It's a fun DIY project. All you need is the magnetic board, some small magnets, and glue. Put a magnet on the bottom or side of each item and attach to the board. Display a mirror nearby and it's your own beauty shop.

MICHELLE PHAN

If you have a lot of makeup, perhaps clear shoeboxes are the way to go. You can sort everything by color and category, like beauty professionals do. Label the front of each shoebox and stack everything in a closet or right out in the open.

YOUR BEAUTY GO BAG

You should always have a beauty go bag packed with essentials and ready to drop in your purse, backpack, or schoolbag. Figure out what items you need throughout the day, and consider emergencies too! A powder compact, a small hand cream, lip balm, lipstick or gloss, antibacterial gel, an adhesive bandage, some feminine products, tissues, a safety pin or two, and some hair elastics will get you through a lot of situations. Don't pack much more than that, or the bag will be too heavy. Toss everything in a makeup bag or pencil case and you're ready for action.

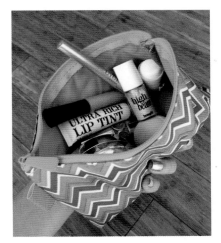

If you can afford it, buy doubles of the products you use most frequently so you can have one set at home and one in your beauty go bag. You'll get out of the house faster knowing you have everything you need already packed and in place.

UNDERNEATH IT ALL

Makeup is empowering and entertaining. I hope that's your takeaway after reading this chapter and learning some of my favorite tricks and tips. But remember, you're beautiful with or without it. I know some of you out there are shaking your heads. You might not believe me now, but one day you'll realize this is true.

And inner beauty? I'd love to devote an entire book to the subject. What's inside your heart, mind, and soul counts more than what's on the outside. Forget lotions, potions, and the latest must-have makeup. The hot item that makes everyone look good? Kindness. Did I mention it's free and one size fits all?

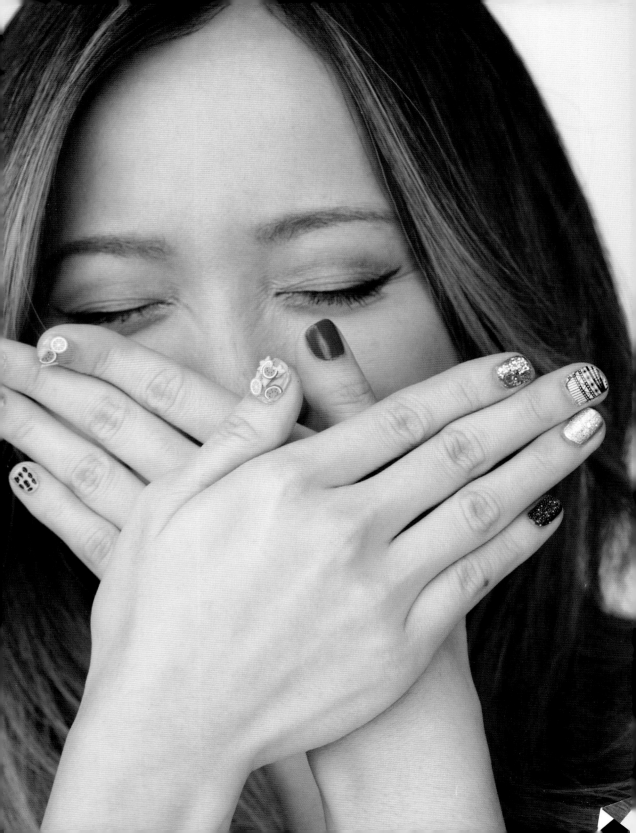

HAIR AND NAILS KNOW-HOW

Obviously, I'm a makeup girl, but I care a lot about hair and nails. It's a package, right? Why have nice makeup and not pay attention to other aspects of being well groomed? My nail obsession clearly dates back to my time at my mom's nail salon. I learned a lot of life lessons hanging out and working there, but I learned practical things too. Such as? Well, you might see me with chipped polish from time to time, but trust me—when I need to, I can give myself a mean manicure!

As for hair, I think my interest stems from the type of hair I was born with—black, thick, and coarse! It's not easy hair to style. Unless I wanted to spend the rest of my life wearing a ponytail, I needed to learn how to deal with it.

I'm going to share a few of the lessons I've learned over the years, as well as some tips and tricks, to help you feel more confident about your hair and nail skills. With some practice and a little know-how, I promise you can become pretty good at being your own hairstylist and manicurist.

YOUR HAIR TYPE AND TEXTURE

Your hair is as personal as your fingerprints. We all know that just by looking at each other. Texturally, my hair is naturally wavy in the back, straight in the front. My hair is also very heavy and coarse, as I mentioned. Instead of flatironing it or curling it each day so it's all one texture, I've learned to live with it. I used to wish my hair was all wavy or all straight, but that wish never came true. You always want what you don't have, especially when it comes to hair. The grass is always greener. Or maybe the hair is always hairier! You know what I mean.

So what kind of hair do you have? Fine, medium, or coarse? Maybe it's straight, wavy, curly, frizzy, or a combination of those qualities? You also can have oily, dry, or normal hair.

Understanding your hair texture and type can help you figure out the best look and cut for you. It's also useful knowledge when it comes to communicating with your hairstylist, which we'll discuss in a little bit.

THE BEST HAIRCUT FOR YOU

Before a single strand on your head gets snipped, you need to do your homework. You can go to a hairstylist and let him or her do what he or she thinks is best, but that might result in disaster. (It's happened to me!) It's better to do some research first and come to the salon armed with magazine tear sheets, photos, and questions.

Go online or flip through some magazines and find celebrities and models with the same hair as you. Don't focus on red carpet pictures. Those are deceiving, because the celebrities have an army of top hairstylists working with them. Instead, look for off-duty photos of celebrities or models that show their true hair type.

When picking your favorites, be realistic. You might love a certain look, but how much styling does it require? How much time are you prepared to invest every morning? Think about your lifestyle. If you're the kind of girl who rolls out of bed and puts her hair in a ponytail every morning, you'll regret a cut with short layers. Or maybe you're considering a short do. Make sure you're emotionally ready for a drastic cut. You don't want to leave the salon in tears! And what about bangs? Bangs are definitely a commitment in terms of time and money because they require frequent trims.

Next, you need to find the stylist who is right for you. Don't ever walk into a salon and let them place you with a random stylist. Again, more potential for disaster. Instead, find out who the best person is for your hair type in your town or city. Ask around, read online reviews—you can even ask strangers. They'll be flattered that you like their hair!

Before you book an appointment, ask the salon how much the stylist costs. A good stylist can be expensive and you don't want any surprises on the day of your haircut. If a certain person is out of reach financially and you can't find someone in your price range, ask if the stylist has an assistant you could book.

Another option is finding a nearby beauty school or a training night at the local salon. You might be able to get your hair cut for free or for a nominal cost. This option might be best if you're the adventurous type, as you could wind up with a look you didn't anticipate!

SALON ETIQUETTE AND TIPPING

It's important that you understand how to talk to your hairstylist. Otherwise you could walk out with a haircut you didn't envision. You should never be afraid to speak up. You won't be hurting your hairstylist's feelings. He or she is a professional, after all. A good hairstylist understands how much emotion is involved, and besides, it's your hair and you are paying for a service.

I vividly remember the worst haircut I ever got. I was fifteen years old. I went in for a trim and left with the shortest hair I've ever had. I knew the stylist was cutting a lot, but I thought perhaps she was layering my hair. It looked terrible, and it was such a waste because all of that hair could have been donated. I left in tears. So speak up when you're in that chair!

A good way to make sure everyone is on the same page is to talk with your stylist pre-haircut. Ask him or her to walk you through what he or she will be doing so you understand what's about to happen. This will allow you to relax during the cut instead of worrying.

This next part is very important. Pay attention as the stylist styles your hair, and don't be afraid to ask questions. Make note of the products and tools used, and take some pictures if you think that will help. (Ask before you start snapping away.)

TIPS ON TIPPING

This can be such a tricky subject at a salon. There are so many people to tip—the person who takes your coat, the assistant who washes your hair, the assistant who helps your stylist, and that's before you even tip your stylist! If you're getting your hair colored too, that doubles everything.

My rule of thumb is 20 percent for the main stylist or colorist (sometimes it's one person who does both). If you are pleased, 15 percent should be the minimum. Ten percent is too low. No one can live on 10 percent tips. Anyone who checks your coat and/or bag should get $1 per item, more if your items are heavy or bulky. As for the assistants, it depends on how much work they did and how much the cut or color was, but $5 to $20 is probably the range. The person who washes your hair should get between $5 and $10. If the person who does your hair owns the salon, you don't have to tip anything.

WASH IT/CONDITION IT

Let's also discuss washing your hair. Do you shampoo too much? Many people do, because washing our hair is a habit we don't even think about. You just do it, right? Even though most shampoo bottles say "wash, rinse, repeat," you don't need to wash your hair twice. That's overdoing it. One shampoo per shower is plenty, unless your hair is really greasy or you haven't washed it in a while.

My next question is, Do you wash your hair every day? You don't necessarily need to. Again, this is something many of us have become accustomed to because of habit and general expectations. If your hair is dry or color treated, you could go a day between washings. Your hair might even benefit from a little break.

How do you wash your hair? Do you throw it up in a bundle and rub a few times, washing everything from roots to ends? The ends of your hair are the driest, so you don't need to shampoo much there. You need to retain as much natural oil at the ends as possible. Instead, focus on your scalp. Then, when you rinse the shampoo from your scalp, let the soapy water run down the length of your hair. That will get the rest of your hair clean enough.

When it comes to choosing a shampoo, look for a product that's compatible with your hair type. You don't necessarily need to spend a lot of money on shampoo because there are so many great drugstore brands.

Did you know there are special shampoos for people who color their hair? I'm a big fan of them. I find they're gentler on your hair than basic shampoo and can help boost color, especially in the case of blond hair or blond highlights. A few salon brands offer purple shampoo—yes, purple!— that prevents blond from going brassy and keeps it on the ashy side, which looks nicer and more natural. The shampoo might seem a little scary though, so be warned! It looks like melted purple crayons. But it's the purple pigment that combats the brassiness. Make sure to follow directions and/or talk to your colorist before using this kind of product.

CONDITIONER

"The more, the better" is my rule when it comes to conditioner. My hair is so coarse, I need two big handfuls before I get out of the shower. I work the conditioner through my hair and leave it in for a few minutes, then I rinse it out.

I do think everyone should use conditioner, but the type you should choose depends on your hair. If you have oily hair, for example, you want a lighter conditioner; dry hair, a heavier one. Be careful if you have fine hair, though. Too much conditioner can weigh down your hair.

How about leave-in conditioner? This is a product you apply in the shower after shampooing but don't wash out. Some people with frizzy or unruly hair love leave-in conditioner because it tames their locks. (But, again, be careful. It can make certain hair types go limp.) Then there is deep conditioner—a great product if you have dry or damaged hair. Apply it after shampooing and leave it in for as long as you need. If you want, hop out of the shower and read a magazine to give the product time to work. After twenty minutes, hop back in and rinse.

DRYING YOUR HAIR

When you get out of the shower or the bath, gently blot your hair with a towel and then wrap it up. Although it's tempting, don't rub your hair dry with the towel. It's damaging to your hair. If you wash your hair at night, don't go to bed with wet hair. You'll wake up with dents in your hair that are almost impossible to remove in the morning! Instead, blow it dry a bit. You don't need it to be bone-dry, but it shouldn't be too damp either.

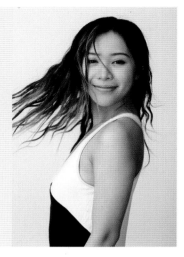

TRUE (OR NOT-SO-TRUE!) COLORS

Chances are, at some point in your life you are going to color your hair. Maybe you do it already; after all, we humans like to mess with the hair nature gave us. And why not? It's fun to change your hair color. Who isn't curious about what it's like to live life as a blonde, brunette, or redhead—or as someone with blue or crimson hair? Today, celebrities and civilians alike rock a rainbow of hues, so it's hard to shock with hair color anymore. Most people don't even bat an eye over an outrageous shade.

Coloring your hair can be fun, empowering, even life changing. I've had a lot of personal experience with hair color, both temporary and permanent. My own hair is dark, dark brown, but I've been going lighter for years. As I write this, I've been experimenting with a rose-gold color that I love. Who knows? I could wake up tomorrow and try something totally different.

TEMPORARY COLOR

It's tough when you make a mistake with permanent hair color. In many cases you can color over it or have a professional colorist repair the dam-

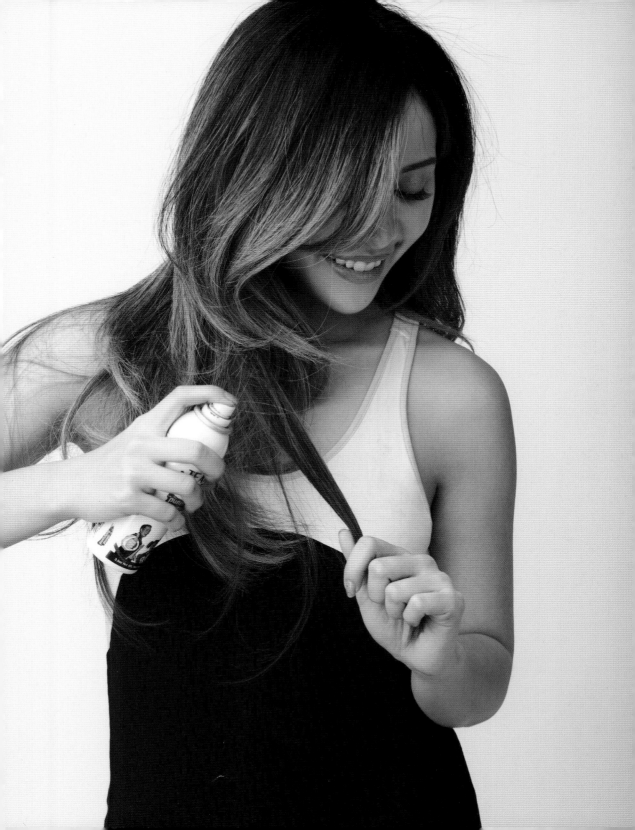

age, but sometimes the only option is to cut it off and let it grow back. We never want you to get to that point!

So let's talk about temporary options. These are great if you like your natural color and just want to play around. Maybe you'll commit to permanent color in the future, maybe not.

One fun option is colored hairspray, which coats your hair with temporary color. It can be a pretty intense look, as the colors are really vivid, but if you want a neon pink streak, a blue ponytail, or a select placement of color, it's a great no-commitment way to get it. You can find these hairsprays at beauty supply shops. Make sure to follow the directions and check out some YouTube tutorials on the subject. Once you use the product, it might take a few washings to get all of the color out of your hair. And be careful if you have light locks! It is possible to stain your hair.

SEMIPERMANENT COLOR

There's an intermediate step between fake and permanent color called semipermanent. It's another way to dip your toe into color without commitment. Stop by your local drugstore or beauty supply shop and find the hair color aisle. Next, look for the boxes of hair color marked semipermanent. You can apply these at home fairly easily and the color will wash out gradually over the course of a few weeks, depending on how frequently you wash your hair.

We're going to talk about coloring your hair at home in a little bit. The rules are the same with permanent and semipermanent color. When buying at-home color, stick to reputable brands. They all have customer hotlines in case you have questions or anything goes wrong.

OMBRÉ

This look burst out of nowhere a few years ago and became the hottest thing in hair color. When I had ombré color, I thought it might be a fad, but it has stuck around. Basically, it is a gradation of color, with the darkest color at your roots and the lightest at the ends. It's a very pretty look, especially on long hair, and is a nice variation on having a single shade or traditional highlights.

With ombré, you're not committing your entire head of hair to a new color—just part of it! There are great at-home ombré kits you can try, or you can have it done by a professional. Chances are you will love the look, but if you don't, you simply color over it.

PERMANENT COLOR

This one is the real deal. If you want to lighten, darken, brighten, or highlight your hair and really go for it, this is the option for you. As with ombré, you can do it at home or visit a professional hair colorist. If you are working with a colorist, discuss what color is best for you. Again, do some research in advance and find the hair color that you think will suit you most. Bring pictures. It will be helpful for your colorist to know what you have in mind.

DIY HAIR COLOR

My mom still colors her own hair to this day, as do millions of women. The best brands have made their at-home hair color kits as easy and foolproof as possible, so you shouldn't be afraid to use them.

Here are a few tips for achieving perfect at-home color:

- Read and follow the directions! Today's kits are the result of decades of trial and error, so don't try to freestyle it.

- Prepare your space in advance with everything you need: towels, timer, reading material. You need to kill a minimum of ten minutes once you finish applying the color.

- Wear your gloves! They come with the color kit for a reason. You don't want stained nails and fingers.

- Make sure you have a flat work surface on which to mix the color.

- Wear an old T-shirt or bathrobe, or have an old towel to put around your shoulders. You don't want to get hair color on anything nice.

- Speaking of towels, don't use your new white towels for this. Have some old or dark towels on hand.

- There's a chance you might splatter color on yourself, the wall, or the sink. You'd be surprised! Have a sponge or wet towel ready to quickly wipe away any splashes.

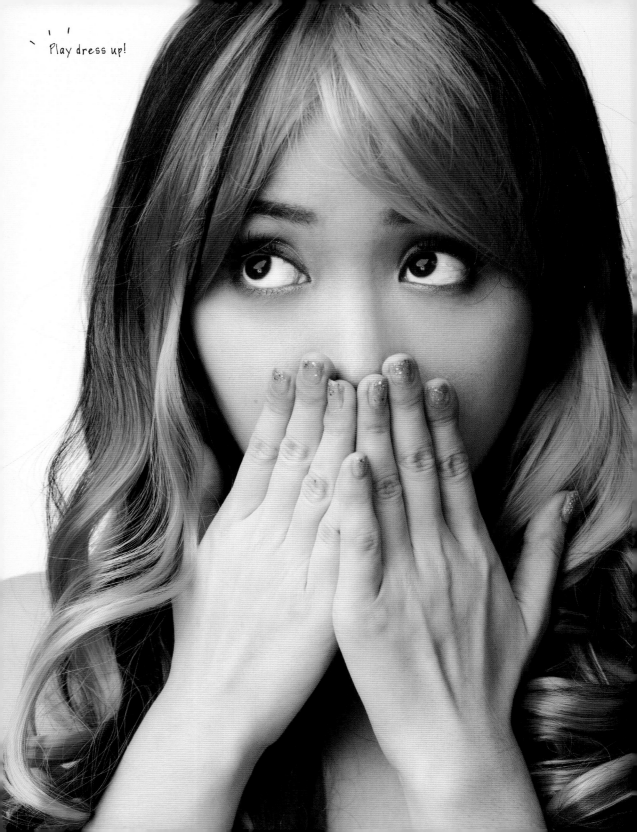

Play dress up!

- Take your time. This isn't a race. You want to schedule enough time to do every step of this process properly, especially if you're a first-timer.

My last piece of advice is not to go too extreme. When you're coloring your hair yourself, it's best to lighten or darken one or two shades above or below your natural color. Anything more dramatic than that—say, blond to black or brunette to cherry red—will probably require a professional's assistance.

WIGS AND HAIRPIECES

If you want to fake it, so many great options exist today, at every price point and in every color. In addition to wigs, there is a whole range of clip-in products—highlights, falls, ponytails, braids, and bangs. If you've seen my videos, you know how much I love a wig. I remember the first time I wore one. I forgot to buy a wig cap, the tight-fitting cap that keeps your real hair out of the way. (It is key to making sure your wig fits well and stays in place.) So I put a pair of pantyhose on my head! I looked like a bank robber, but it did the trick. If you are going to wear a wig, you should wind your wet hair around your head and bobby-pin it to your scalp, then put on the wig cap. Get your hair as flat as possible.

My whole look transformed as soon as I put on the wig. You should definitely wear a wig once in your life, whether it's a crazy one or a serious color, just to see how it changes your entire appearance. You'll be shocked. My current favorite wig? It's a rainbow one that makes me look like a galactic mermaid. Wearing it is so much fun.

The most realistic, and expensive, wig and hairpiece options are made from real hair. They're so good you'll even fool yourself while wearing them. As for synthetic hair, some pieces can look surprisingly natural. Others, though, won't fool anyone! They're more like Barbie hair than the real stuff—but that's okay. Sometimes it's fun to fake it.

Check your local beauty supply shop or look online for a selection of hairpieces. If you're trying to perfectly match your actual hair color, you're better off buying something in person. Step outside with the hairpiece (with permission, of course!) and a mirror and make sure it blends in natural light.

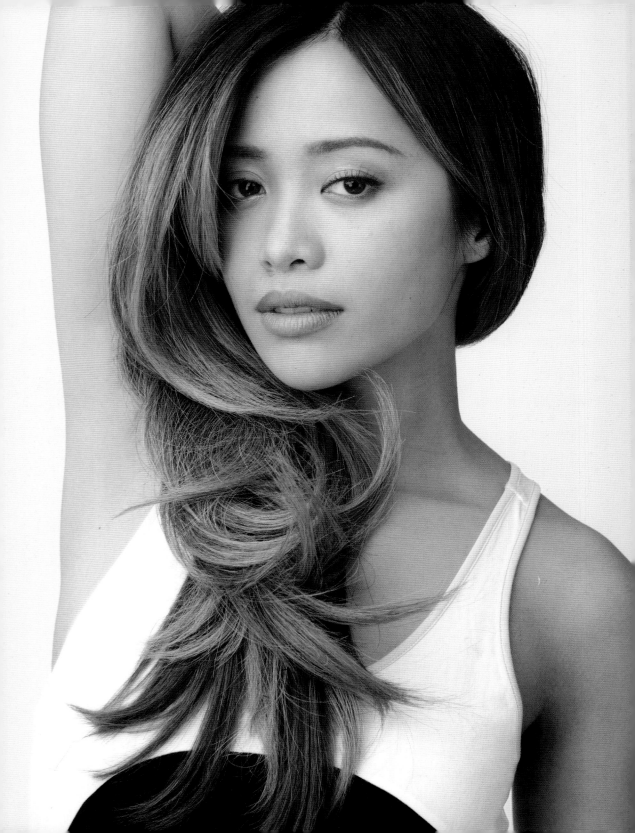

ALL-NATURAL HAIR TREATMENTS

You can't beat Mother Nature when it comes to beauty products. A few of my favorite hair treatments come from the health food store. Take coconut oil. I apply it to the ends of my hair, where it's driest. Just remember to wash your hair in the morning!

Have you ever used a vinegar rinse on your hair? It's a great way to remove hair product residue and restore shine. And don't worry, the vinegar won't make your hair smell. Take some white vinegar or apple cider vinegar and put half a cup to a full cup in a squeeze bottle or old shampoo bottle. Dilute it with an equal amount of water. (The total amount of liquid necessary depends on the length of your hair.) Wash your hair, then douse it with the vinegar solution. Work it through with your fingers and rinse with warm water. Follow with a bit of conditioner. So simple.

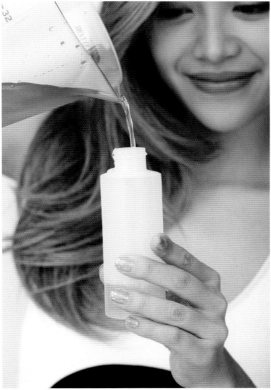

DO YOUR DO!

Don't you wish a stylist could come to your house every morning and do your hair? That would be a dream come true. Until then, we have to be our own stylists. But that's okay. There are lots of tools, tricks, and products that can help you replicate what a professional does.

QUICK CHANGE—SWITCH UP YOUR PART

This is the easiest way to update your look. There's no commitment and you don't need any product or expert assistance. At the most, you'll need a comb. How do you currently part your hair? A middle part can look sweet and innocent. Think Alice in Wonderland or Snow White. Or it can look very cool in a chic hippie kind of way. Side parts can provide a variety of looks as well. A severe side part can be sexy or retro—think Jessica Rabbit. I'm not a huge fan of the zigzag part. It looks a bit weird having this perfect zigzag on your head. Mess it up a bit and it will look much better. In fact, a messy off-center part is the most contemporary looking.

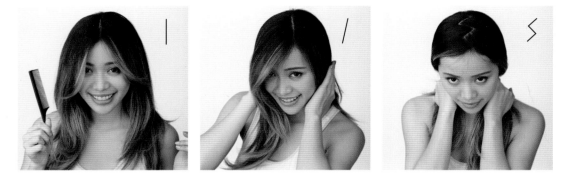

TOOL TIME
Here are my go-to tools:

- Curling iron
- Flat bristle brush
- Hair dryer
- Round brush
- Flatiron

Curling Iron

I use this tool the most. With a little experimentation, it's relatively easy to master.

First, you need to figure out the appropriate barrel size. The barrel is the part of the curling iron that heats up and gives you the actual curl. Curling irons come in different sizes, from half an inch to two inches. Smaller barrels result in tighter curls; larger barrels create looser curls.

If you are new to curling irons, before you buy anything watch some tutorials to figure out the barrel size that's best for the look you want to achieve. Once you have your new curling iron, give yourself a weekend to watch some more videos, sit in front of a mirror, and experiment. You really want to find videos of people using curling irons on themselves, as opposed to stylists demonstrating on models. The movements and techniques are different when you are doing your own hair.

When you're browsing YouTube, you'll probably come across the famous video of the girl whose lock of hair came right off when she was using a curling iron. Yes, it is possible to burn your hair off with a curling iron! There are a few things you can do to avoid any similar disasters. First, make sure your hair is completely dry when using a curling iron or flatiron. Second, check the heat setting on the appliance. Leave the highest setting to the professionals. If you're using the appliance for the first time, start with the lowest setting. If you need more heat, you can turn it up. Third, don't leave the appliance in one place with your hair in it for too long. For curling irons, five to seven seconds per one-inch section should be enough time. If not, perhaps you're trying to curl too much hair. Try thinner sections. As for flatirons, they are meant to be moved over a section of hair, not left in place. Keep it moving!

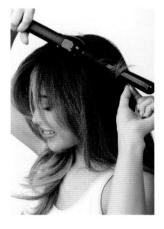

This last tip goes without saying, but you should always read the instruction manual before using any appliance.

How do *I* use a curling iron? I actually use two different ones—a half-inch barrel and a one-and-a-half inch one. Having different curl sizes gives me a more natural look than one uniform curl size. I section off my hair (you can use clips if your hair is really thick), then take a one-inch piece and wrap it around the first barrel. The next piece goes around the second barrel, and so on. After I do my entire head of hair, I gently brush out the curls from root to tip once with my flat bristle brush. (Starting at the bottom and working your way up each section to your scalp, bit by bit, will remove too much of the curl.)

Hair Dryer

This might seem like a basic tool, but you can achieve a variety of looks with a hair dryer. You can use it as-is to dry your hair for a natural look. You can add a diffuser to the end of your blow dryer if you have curly hair. (A diffuser literally diffuses the hot air, which makes curly hair less frizzy and doesn't break up the curl as much as normal blow-drying.) And, of course, you can use a hair dryer to give yourself a blowout.

I'll confess—I'm not very good at blowouts. I have too much hair and it

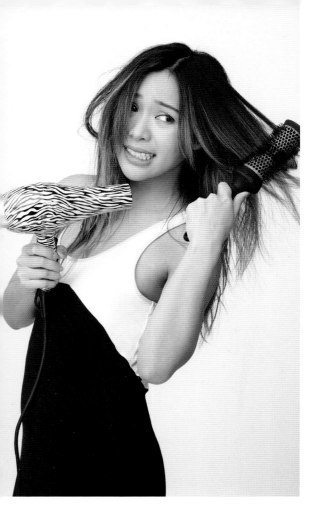

takes me forever to do. That's why I love a professional blowout, and I'm in awe when I meet anyone who is great at a DIY blowout.

If you love the look of a blowout, you should definitely learn how to do it. To get started, section off your hair and clip the top layer to the top of your head. Next, have your hair dryer and round brush ready. Starting at the bottom layer of hair and working with one-inch sections, wrap your hair around the brush and hold the blow dryer right near the hair. (Don't let the blow dryer touch your hair.) Move the brush and the blow dryer together from root to ends. You want to pull on your hair somewhat to get it as straight as possible. Don't pull so hard that you yank it out of your head! But you definitely want and need some tension there. Remove the clips and do the top layer once the bottom is done.

Now, you can do all sorts of variations depending on the final look you're going for. Do you want it really sleek and flat, or do you want some body with a bit of movement at the ends? It's going to require a bit of experimentation and playing around, but take the time to figure it out. You've got a lifetime of doing your hair ahead of you!

MAKE YOUR BLOWOUT LAST You can extend the life of your blowout with a good dry shampoo. This lifesaver comes in powder or aerosol form. Hold the bottle or can about ten inches away from your roots, spray, and then brush it out. The dry shampoo soaks up oil and adds fragrance, so the blowout looks and smells fresh. But you can only do this for so long! Don't try to overextend your blowout. Your hair will get stinky if you don't wash it after a while, no matter how much dry shampoo you use.

MICHELLE PHAN

Flatiron

A flatiron is a great tool if you want that sleek, straight look. If you were born with straight hair and want it stick straight, you can run your flat-iron through it. If you give yourself a blowout, you can use your flatiron as the final touch to get the hair just so.

Follow the same rules I gave you for using a curling iron. Read the directions first, make sure your hair is completely dry, don't use the hottest setting, work with one-inch sections of hair, and keep the iron moving. Don't leave it in place. You could burn off your hair! I know I told you all of this already, but it's worth repeating.

THE BRAID PARADE

Braids are a great break from boring everyday hair. Two types of braids in particular—the French braid and the fishtail braid—look so beautiful and are easy to do on yourself.

A French braid is much simpler than it looks. If you know how to do a basic braid, you can master the French braid. First, decide where you want the braid to be. Next, take a portion of hair from the top or front of where the braid will begin and divide it into three sections. Start braiding. You know the braiding pattern: over, under, over, under, over, under. Well, each time you make the over movement, incorporate some extra hair into the section. Remember to keep everything tight. When you get to the bottom of your hair, secure with an elastic. Practice makes perfect with French braiding, so play around until you get the hang of it. I know people who can French-braid their own hair without even looking in a mirror, so practice while you're watching TV. Next, you can experiment with different types of French braids. You can have one big braid down the back of your head, or you can have a braid on each side that meets in the back. Either pin the braids into place, or take the braids and make one larger braid down the back of your head. There are so many variations.

The fishtail braid is a beautiful braid that slightly resembles a fishbone or a herringbone pattern. Start by dividing your hair into two sections. Let's call them Sections #1 and #2. Take a small section of hair from the outside of Section #1, pull it across Section #1, and incorporate the small piece into Section #2. Now take a small section of hair from the outside of Section #2, pull it across Section #2, and incorporate the small piece into

Section #1. Repeat from the beginning and keep going to the bottom of your hair. As you move each piece of hair, keep pulling tight. When you finish, secure your hair with an elastic.

Now that you've learned a few tricks for your hair, let's fast forward to our fingers and our toes!

BEAUTIFUL HANDS AND FEET

Having nicely maintained hands and feet tells the world you are a well-groomed person. But, more important, it makes you feel good about yourself. I swear! When your nails and toes look kind of gnarly, it seriously bums you out. Pretty toes and fingernails, on the other hand, will make you smile. Especially your hands. After all, you probably see them all day as you work on your computer, write, drive, and do other activities.

In this section, we're going to talk about the steps you can take to have nice-looking hands and feet. You need to get a few tools and dedicate some time to the process, but it will be worth it. After all, these are investments in you!

NAILS: THE ULTIMATE ACCESSORY

Any time I see someone with unpolished nails, I think, "What a missed opportunity!" The whole nail category is so much fun today. When I was younger, there was no such thing as nail stickers, and nail art hadn't exploded yet. Nails are truly a canvas for your creativity, and so much less permanent or serious than experimenting with hair, clothing, or makeup. Piercing one nail and hanging a charm on it is certainly not the same as piercing your nose or eyebrow, now, is it? One you can change up tomorrow, and the other you're kind of stuck with! It's the same with nail color versus hair color. You can have a fun ombré rainbow across all ten nails, but do the same to your hair? Well, you can, but it's a thousand times more work and commitment.

I'm not sure why I love nails as much as I do. Maybe it's all that time spent in my mom's salon, listening to the customers and helping out. Or the fact that I love art and painting so much. After all, each nail is a mini portable canvas.

KNOW YOUR NAIL TYPE

As with hair and skin, you have a nail type specific to you. Some people can grow their nails long and strong; others have weak nails that don't grow very much or brittle nails that break easily. Just as with your hair, you can take specific vitamins and minerals to help strengthen your nails and make them grow faster. Ask for a recommendation at your local health food or vitamin store.

THE DIY MANICURE

Anyone can master nail maintenance, I promise! With a little bit of practice, you can get very good at doing your own manicures. I'm going to walk you through it.

One note: If you want to do a proper manicure, make sure to schedule enough time. This isn't an activity you should rush through. Plus, you need to factor in time for your polish to dry. If done properly, your manicure should last all week. Just remember to wear gloves when doing any housework, especially when washing the dishes. That is the number one manicure killer!

Your Nail Shape

Before any clipping, filing, or painting takes place, you need to know what nail shape you want. The options are pointy, round, oval, square, or squoval (a combination of square and oval, basically a square shape with the corners softened). You also need to decide what length—short, medium, or long.

I'm not a fan of super-long nails. If you're a celebrity with a manicurist on call all the time, a long nail is great and looks cool in photos and music videos. But in real life they just get in the way, not to mention all that dirt and bacteria that gets trapped underneath. Yuck.

The Tools You Need

Here are the basic items I would like you to have on hand for a DIY manicure:

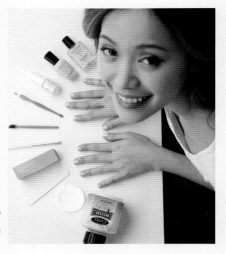

- Nail polish remover
- Cotton balls or pads
- Nail clipper or scissor
- Nail file
- Nail buffer
- Cuticle clipper
- Cuticle oil
- Orange stick (This skinny stick is not orange, just FYI. It's named that because it used to be made from orangewood!)
- Clear top coat/base coat (Buy a combination product rather than spending money on a separate top coat and base coat.)
- Nail polish

Shape and Smooth Your Nails

Always start by washing your hands. Then, to get started, remove any old polish with your nail polish remover and cotton. Next, use your nail clipper or scissor to cut your nails to the desired shape and length. I prefer clipping, and only on dry nails. Wet nails are too soft and can be damaged by clipping. Clipping or cutting will leave sharp edges, so use your nail file to smooth down any jagged bits. At the same time, you want to file your nail into the desired shape, so keep that in mind. Be gentle when filing; don't saw away at your nail like it's a piece of wood.

PUT DOWN YOUR NAIL CLIPPER!
Do not clip your nails in public or in the office! So many people do this and I never understand why. Serious grooming should be done in the privacy of your own home.

Next, use your nail buffer to buff the top, side, and edge of each nail. If you're not familiar with buffing, it's a technique that smoothes your nails and leaves a subtle satiny finish. You can buy a nail buffer in any drugstore or beauty supply shop. When buffing, apply a bit of pressure, but be gentle. It's your nails we're talking about, not a big piece of furniture or a car!

Buffing preps your nails nicely for polish because it leaves a smooth surface. If you're a natural kind of girl, buffing is a great substitution for nail polish. Natural or not, keep reading! We have more work to do on our nails.

Your Cuticles

Now it's time to tend to your cuticles. This is the skin that runs along the bottom and sides of your nails. Regular cuticle maintenance will reduce the number of pesky hangnails you get. (If you do get a hangnail, please don't pick at it! Try to ignore it until you can get home and clip it properly.) The idea of cutting your own cuticles might seem scary, but we're not actually cutting the entire cuticle. We're just tending to any rough bits or pieces or anything that can develop into a hangnail.

> ### DRY SKIN = MORE HANGNAILS
> If you have dry cuticles, remember to moisturize your hands after you wash them and apply your cuticle oil or a special cuticle cream before you go to bed. That should help alleviate any dryness and cut down on the hangnails. And, as mentioned earlier, wear gloves when doing housework. Cleaning products tend to be harsh and can further dry out your skin.

When cutting, just remember to go slow and work in very small, almost bitsy areas. Never attempt to cut a large area at once.

Before you cut a single thing, however, take some cuticle oil and massage it into your cuticles. Next, use your orange stick to carefully push your cuticles back. You'll see any bits that need to be clipped. If the cutting process totally scares you, go to a good manicurist first and watch how she or he does it. Then it might be easier to replicate at home.

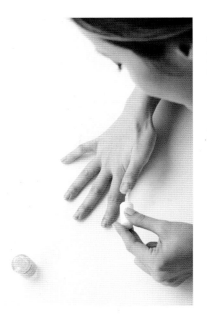

Base Coat

After tending to your cuticles, use your polish remover and cotton to wipe your nail beds. This will remove any residue from the cuticle oil and help your nail polish last longer. Take your base/top coat combo and paint a thin layer on each nail. This will protect your nail bed from discoloration and extend the life of your manicure.

If your nails are weak, you can use a nail strengthener in place of a base coat. Whichever you use, let it dry completely before moving on to the next step. Clear nail polish only takes a minute or so to dry.

POLISH MAKES PERFECT

The secret to a perfect polish job is practice, practice, practice. You can experiment on someone else's nails, but it's not the same as doing your own. After all, if you're a righty, for example, you can do someone else's entire polish job with your right hand. But you need to be ambidextrous when doing your own. It takes some trial and error to get the hang of it.

You might think all nail polish is the same, but it's not. Formulas can be very different. Some are thin and meant to be layered. Others are thick and can do the job in one coat. Some are more long lasting; some chip easily. Here are some of the different payoffs and textures:

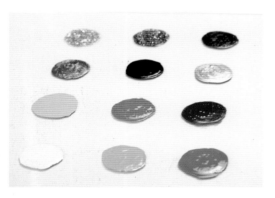

- Sheer polish is a light wash of color and the most natural looking of all polishes. This can look different in the bottle than it does on the nail, so test the color before you buy. When a sheer color chips, it's not terribly noticeable, so you can push the lifespan of a sheer manicure a bit longer than with other polish types.

- Opaque polish is a solid color you can't see through and the best choice when you are wearing a statement color.

- Glitter nail polish has actual pieces of glitter suspended in it.

- Frosted/shimmer/pearl polish has added ingredients such as mica to give it that particular appearance.

- High-shine formulas provide a more glossy finish.

- Matte formulas have no shine. Rather than buy an entire bottle of matte polish, you can turn regular polish into matte very easily. Bring a pot of water to a boil. Paint your nails, and while the polish is still wet, wave them above the steam a few times. (Do this quickly. Don't leave your hands over the water too long or you could burn yourself!) Something about the water and the wet polish causes it to dry to a matte finish. Just think. You can make ramen and mattify your nails at the same time!

What I said about polish formulas is true about nail polish brushes too. Some brushes are thick and flat, some are skinny, some are slightly curved. You might want to try a few different brands and see which you find the easiest to maneuver.

If you're new to the world of nail polish, ask around, read reviews, or check out nail blogs to find out what polishes are the best ones. There are so many great ones, you can get lost for hours!

Chipped Nail Polish

So many people rock this look today—supermodels, movie stars, beauty editors. It used to be a super-edgy look, but now it's almost mainstream. In the past, it was a beauty no-no to have chipped nails; now people are more relaxed about it. That said, there's a fine line between looking cool and looking lazy. Don't cross that line with super-chipped nails.

Polish Application

Choose the polish you want to use and apply one coat, not too thick and not too thin. Let it dry and apply a second coat. Let that dry. If you made any mistakes with your polish, wrap a tiny piece of cotton or tissue around the top of your orange stick and dip the stick into your nail polish remover. Rub the top of the stick over any polish that needs to be removed or cleaned up.

For the final step, apply your base/top coat. Let that dry and you are done! How great do your nails look?

> ### DISCOLORED NAILS
> A quick note about discoloration. Even with a base coat underneath, your nails can get discolored if you wear dark polishes, such as black or purple, especially for extended periods of time. Those shades can turn your nail bed yellowish. It's not dangerous; it's just not pretty. What can you do about it? You'll need to stop wearing dark colors and let your nails grow out, or learn to live with it.

SPECIALTY NAILS

The French Manicure

The traditional French features a white tip and a sheer pink or natural base. No one is quite sure why it's called a French manicure. No one in France calls it that, because it's an American invention!

The pink-and-white French is a bit played out, but I love a French in different color combinations. You can experiment and use your favorite colors: hot pink and black, red and sky blue, or lilac and gray, for example. Or try this: Do one base color and make each tip a different color. There's no reason you need to stick to the original. Have fun with it.

The Moon Manicure

Do you know what the moon of your nail is? Take a look at your naked thumbnail and examine the bottom third or quarter. Do you notice how the base is curved and paler than the rest of your nail? That part is called the moon. It might be visible on all of your nails or just a few of them.

This is the inspiration for a very cool kind of manicure in which the moon is painted with one color or with clear polish while the rest of the nail gets a second color. It looks really romantic and gives the illusion of long nails and fingers. Believe it or not, the moon manicure dates back to the 1930s and '40s!

Nail Art

You can take nail art as far as you want. You can make simple squiggles and dots with a nail pen, apply decals, or go wild with 3-D nail art like the Japanese do. It's really mind-boggling what the Japanese are doing with this beauty category. Google "3-D Japanese nail art" and you won't believe it. Hello Kitty, bows, cherry blossoms, cupcakes, all rising off the nail like mini sculptures.

Nail Stickers

These are fun for people who want something more interesting than basic polish. I use a lot of nail stickers because I'm constantly filming different videos, sometimes up to three a day, and I need different nail looks for each tutorial. It would be impossible to polish my nails three times a day! Not to mention how bad it would be for my nails to use nail polish remover that frequently. (Nail polish remover can dry out your nails.)

You also can find stickers that look just like basic nail polish. If you're pressed for time or aren't good at painting your nails, you'll love this option.

Before using your nail stickers, apply a base coat and let it dry. You should always have a protective layer between your nail bed and nail color, nail art, or nail stickers.

To apply, take your packet of stickers. You're going to start with the pinkie on your left hand and work across all your fingers. Find the sticker with the shape and size closest to that of your pinkie nail. Trim the sides if necessary to make it fit perfectly. (We'll worry about any excess on the top in just a minute.) Remove the backing and apply it to your nail, stretching it slightly so that it covers the entire nail. Your thumb is a good tool for doing this. Next, use a pair of nail scissors or a nail file to remove any excess sticker along the top of the nail. Sometimes the sticker kits come with a special file you can use. Repeat on all your other nails.

The process is not going to be easy the first time you do it, but with some practice it will become quite simple. You'll be able to apply new stickers in less than ten minutes—way less time than it takes for nail polish to dry!

Gels and Acrylics

These are two types of artificial nails that are literally sculpted right on top of your nail. They're great for people who can't grow their own nails or who need a manicure that will be bulletproof for a few weeks. I had gels once. I was about to do a world tour for Lancôme and I wanted something that would last the duration of the trip, so I got purple gel nails. I was amazed how much I could do with them without worrying about chips or breakage.

The process can be long and expensive and you want to find a talented technician. Once you get acrylics or gels, your work isn't over, however. You will need to return to the salon for what's called a "fill-in." Because your nails are always growing, eventually you'll see the area of new growth at the base of your nails. You need to get that area filled in with the acrylic or gel formula. It's not so noticeable if you chose a natural nail polish color. But if you have a strong or bold color, it's very noticeable.

The biggest difference between gels and acrylics is appearance. Acrylics are thick and less flexible, gels are thinner and more flexible. I find gels to be more attractive and natural looking, but each type has its fans.

BEST FOOT FORWARD

I love pretty toes. There's something about a nicely maintained foot that is so lovely and makes you feel better about everything. Truly!

There's nothing more pampering than a salon pedicure, but I've gotten pretty good at doing my own version of it at home. It's a fun, relaxing thing to do for yourself. Here's how.

DIY PEDICURE

Just as with manicures, do this when you have some time to yourself. A proper pedicure will take at least an hour once you factor in drying time.

The tools you need

There are some basic tools you should have on hand for a DIY pedicure:

- Nail polish remover
- Cotton balls or pads
- Nail clipper or scissor
- Nail file
- Large bowl filled with warm water
- One lime, cut in half. Reserve one half and cut the other half into slices.
- Cuticle oil
- Orange stick
- Cuticle clipper
- Foot file
- Towel
- Body lotion
- Toe separators
- Clear top coat/base coat
- Nail polish

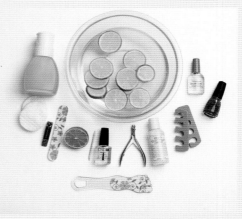

The first step is to remove any old polish with your nail polish remover and cotton. Next, clip and file your toenails. The best shape for toenails is square, following the natural shape that already exists. You might need to file the corners down slightly if they are too sharp, but you don't want rounded-edge toenails.

Next, fill your bowl with warm water and the lime slices. You'll love how nice it smells. Put your feet in the bowl, let them soak a bit—at least five minutes—then take the half a lime and start scrubbing your feet with it. Get your toes and everything. It really refreshes and cleans your feet. Put your feet back in the water. Once the skin has softened somewhat, use your orange stick to gently push your cuticles back. If they need extra love, apply some oil, then gently clip anywhere the skin is ragged or rough, or needs to be trimmed.

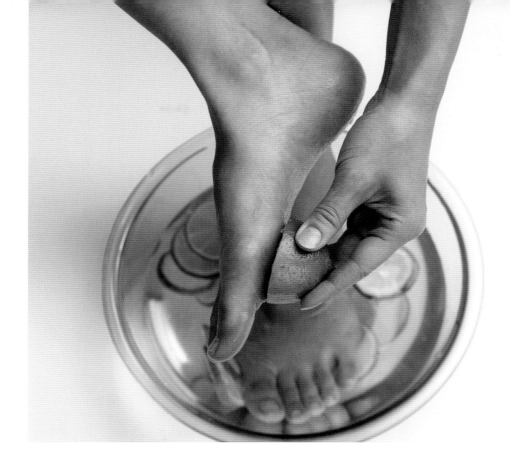

Calluses

Let's talk about calluses for a minute. These are areas of thickened skin on our feet that occur because of friction from high heels or ill-fitting footwear. Calluses can appear on the balls of our feet, the sides, the heels, and even the toes. What can you do about them? Well, you can cut or clip them, but I advise leaving that to the experts, like a podiatrist or excellent manicurist. Instead, invest in a foot file, those implements that look like cheese graters, but for your feet! Keep it in the shower and use it every few days. Be gentle when using it. Don't grate your feet raw!

If you have calluses, during your DIY pedicure you can gently file your feet after you deal with your cuticles.

Primed for Paint

Rinse your feet one last time, then dry them with the towel. Take some body lotion or cream and moisturize your feet. Really massage the product into your heels, toes, everywhere. Next, take the nail polish remover and wipe your nail beds. If you have anything greasy on your nail beds, your polish won't adhere.

Take your toe separators (they're funny looking, aren't they?) and insert them between your toes. You also can use a paper towel that you've folded into one long strip. The idea here is just to keep your toes away from one another so your nail polish doesn't smear. Just wind the paper between your toes, making sure it doesn't touch your nails.

Next, follow the polish directions in the manicure section. You need a base coat, two coats of polish, and a top coat.

As for the polish you choose, I love bright colors for my toes. Something about looking down and seeing a cheery color makes me happy. Otherwise, you can never go wrong with a good nude color on your toes. Let each coat dry well before applying the next. Once everything is completely dry, you are done! Don't your feet look great?

BABY-SOFT FEET

Let's show our feet a little extra TLC. Next time you're sitting around watching TV or a movie, take some petroleum jelly or thick lotion and slather it on your feet. Throw on some thick cotton socks and leave them on for an hour or two. You can even sleep in them. The next day, your feet will be buttery soft, like a baby's. You should try to do this at least once a week.

Don't do this immediately after a pedicure. You don't want the socks to smear the polish. Make sure your toenails are completely dry before putting on socks or shoes.

BANISH THE BIRD CLAWS!

I don't have many hard-and-fast beauty "rules." If you love something or a certain look, I always say go for it. Except when it comes to long toenails. This is my number one beauty pet peeve. There is nothing pretty or interesting about long toenails, especially with open-toe shoes or sandals! They are like falcon claws. Clip those things!

Also, you should never let your toenails get so long that they dig into each other. Trim them before it gets to that point. It's for your own benefit.

NAVIGATING THE NAIL SALON

There's nothing nicer than going to a nail salon and being pampered. It's great if you can afford it or want to treat yourself. At the same time, there's nothing worse than coming home from the salon with an infection or some other problem. You need to be smart about the salon you choose. They're not all created equal.

The first thing you want to look for is cleanliness. Is everything spotless? How are the tools maintained? Are they sterilizing everything? Is the sterilizer out in the open so you can see? (If you want to be really careful, you can bring your own set of tools. A lot of women do that.) If not, inquire how they keep everything sterilized. If the salon looks sketchy or dirty in any way, walk out. It's not worth it. You also can check the bathroom. That's my test for salons and restaurants. If the bathrooms are clean, chances are the place is clean too. If the bathrooms aren't clean, well . . .

Also, how are the manicurist's own hands? Are his or her nails trimmed and clean? That's a good sign. Dirty, unkempt nails are a terrible sign. If you see that, excuse yourself and go.

Last, be careful about bargains. Sometimes things are cheap for a reason. You get what you pay for.

If you have any doubts about a salon, just leave. Or just ask for a polish change. Don't let them file, trim, or cut anything. Remember, this is supposed to be a relaxing experience for you. If you spend the whole time worried about potential problems, what's the point?

YOU'VE NAILED IT

Do you feel like you've been to beauty school? Hopefully, you're more confident about your hair and nails and your ability to do them yourself. Hair, on the other hand, can take some time. But make that time investment in mastering your mane. Practice, experiment, watch some tutorials. It will be worth it. Of course, there will be bad hair days—they happen to all of us—but remember, that's why the universe created hats!

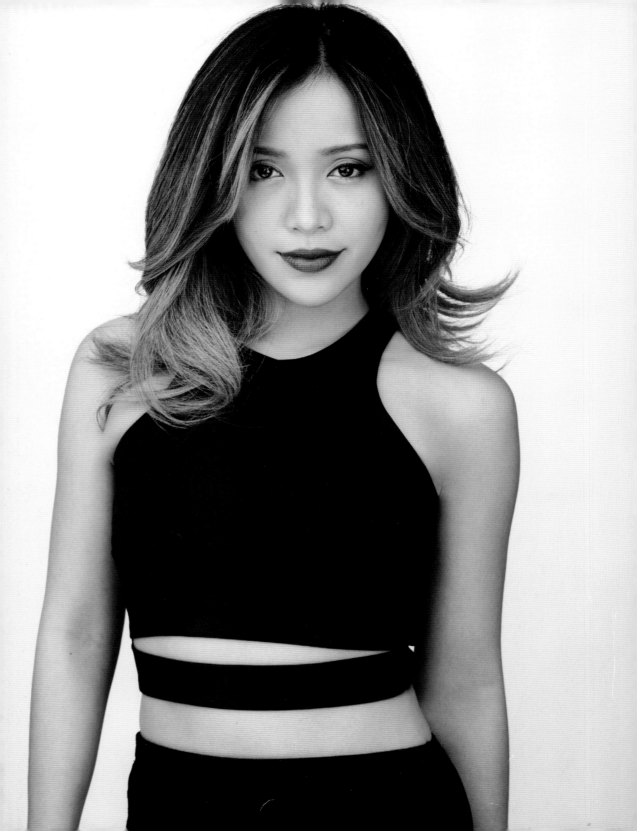

FASHION TIPS AND TRICKS

Fashion is such an intensely personal thing. What we wear conveys who we are, what we like, and how creative we are. People always say, "Don't judge a book by its cover," but the world *does* judge us by our appearances. In a way, we're programmed to be like this. Look at nature! A bumblebee seeks out only certain flowers. Male birds have flashier feathers than female birds to help them attract their mates. When you're picking out an apple, don't you gravitate toward the shiniest one? You don't pick the rotten piece of fruit.

That said, I don't think the shoes on your feet or the clothes on your back have anything to do with the person you are. I'd like to see people judged by more important things—how kind they are and what they contribute to humanity, for example. Yet, I do think how you dress can convey a sense of respect—or disrespect—for others. And you know respect is one of my big issues! So in this chapter, I'm going to share some guidelines to help you put your best self forward and navigate the often-tricky world of what to wear.

I also happen to love fashion, and I believe it's a great form of self-expression, so we'll talk about having a sense of style and what that means. You don't have a sense of style? Are you sure? In that case, I'll help you find yours.

I truly believe everyone can be stylish. It has nothing to do with where you live, how much money you have, or how trendy your clothes are. It's about looking your best in a timeless, classy way that reflects the real you.

WHAT IS STYLE?

That's a good question. According to the dictionary, style is a manner of doing something. In this case, it's how you wear your clothes and what kind of image you project. It's what you evoke as a person. Do you dress up every day in an outfit you planned the night before? Or do you roll out of bed and throw on your sweats and a T-shirt? Do you look sharp, sexy, casual, or comfy? There's also your body language. Do you stand up straight, head held high? Or do you shrink into yourself and try to hide? Your body language plus your fashion choices equals your style.

Let's take it a step further. Is your style personal or impersonal? If you go into a store and buy what you see on a mannequin, you were styled by that brand. There's not much thought behind it. It might be beautiful, and you probably look good, but what does it say about you? If you just wear what your friends wear, that's impersonal too. You tell your own story through your clothing. What story are your clothes telling about you?

> **THERE ARE FOUR KINDS OF PEOPLE WHEN IT COMES TO FASHION. WHICH ONE ARE YOU?**
>
> 1. Comfort is your number one priority. You don't really care what you wear.
> 2. You want to look nice without putting too much thought into it.
> 3. You do care and you plan out your outfits.
> 4. You are an individual who marches to his or her own fashion beat.

THE TRUTH ABOUT TRENDY

Today, it's so easy to confuse being trendy with being stylish. They are not the same. Being trendy means you only wear the latest things—a certain shoe shape, hemline, designer, type of jeans, color, pattern, design. You know what I'm talking about. Being stylish, on the other hand, is looking great, but in an indefinable way. A stylish person looks pulled together and projects a certain sense of confidence. You can be a stylish punk rocker, you can be a stylish preppy, or you can be something in between.

When you're trendy, people notice what you're wearing first. When you're stylish, they notice *you*.

Now, don't get me wrong. I don't want to be a buzzkill about trends, because they can be a lot of fun. After all, trends keep things fresh, new, and exciting and help push fashion forward. Without trends, who knows what we'd look like today? But there's a difference between being a trendsetter and being a trend follower. The first one is way more interesting!

If you want to work a few trendy pieces into your wardrobe, go ahead, but don't spend a lot of money on them. Hit a lower-priced store that specializes in that kind of clothing.

LOGOMANIA

Speaking of trendy, I know some of you love logos. You wear them on your bags, your clothes, your shoes—you can't get enough of them. If you want to carry or wear something with a logo, that's cool. Just don't overdo it. Wearing logos head to toe is a no-no. One logo at a time is fine.

HOW TO BUILD A WARDROBE

You don't need a huge clothing collection to consider what you have a "wardrobe." It's not something restricted to movie stars and fashion editors with walk-in closets. The idea of a wardrobe is that each item of clothing you own has a purpose, goes with your other clothes, and is organized properly. There are benefits to approaching what you wear in this manner:

- Less scrambling to get dressed and out of the house because you're more organized.

- No standing in front of your closet and saying, "I have nothing to wear."

- No more money-wasting impulse purchases. How many times have you bought something and realized it doesn't go with anything you already own? That won't happen again.

TAKE INVENTORY

We're dividing this activity into two parts. First, take inventory of your daily clothing requirements. Here's an example. Let's say you are an assistant at an office that you drive to. You jog, you walk your dog, you go dancing with your friends on the weekends, and you do a little online dating. What clothing do you need for all of these activities? And don't forget clothes for hanging around the house and sleeping. Make sure to include basics, like undergarments and socks, too. Write down what clothes you need each day. Add a section for special-occasion clothing. Do you have a lot of weddings, parties, or family functions coming up? You should always have one nice dress or suit on hand for these events or any last-minute functions.

Next, I want you to go through every article of clothing you own. Pick a weekend or day off and gather everything together. Go ahead and pile it on your bed or somewhere clean. Leave your shoes on the floor and put your accessories on a table or desk. Now look at the list you made of your daily clothing requirements and divide your clothes accordingly. Make one pile for your main activity (work or school), one for each hobby/sport/exercise, one for special occasions, one for dates/nights out, etc. Next, divide each of those piles into the clothes you wear the most and the clothes you wear the least.

If you wear all of your clothes, you get a gold star and can skip ahead. If you have unworn clothing in your closet, keep reading.

YOUR UNLOVED CLOTHING

Let's talk about the clothes you don't wear. Pick up each piece and ask yourself why you don't wear it. If it doesn't fit, what's the problem? Too big or too small? Did you buy it hoping you would be a different size one day? If you're working toward a certain goal regarding your size, that's fine. Keep the article of clothing. You can hang it in a special place in your closet until you are ready for it. If you're not working toward a goal, put that clothing in the good-bye pile. (You're going to take it to a charity, swap it with a friend, or sell it on eBay.) You want to focus on clothes for the person you are today, right this very minute!

How about pieces you just don't like or that are unflattering? Those go straight to the good-bye pile. What about items you like but that don't go with anything? Let's call them your unloved pieces. There are two options. If you have the money to go shopping, buy something that goes with them. If you can't shop right now, put your unloved clothes in the good-bye pile.

There's no use keeping them around to remind you of the things you're missing in your wardrobe! Try to sell or swap them so it's not a total waste of money.

THE MISSING PIECES

Maybe you have too many basics and not enough statement pieces, or vice versa. Maybe you don't have enough accessories or the right undergarments. See what you need to make everything come together. Again, if you can afford to shop, go ahead and fill in the blanks in your wardrobe. If you can't afford to shop, put together a wish list in order of importance. You can add pieces as you can afford them or find them on sale.

YOUR PERSONAL LOOK BOOK

Now you're going to put together some looks. Pretend you're a fashion editor and have some fun with this. We're talking head-to-toe looks, so don't forget your shoes and accessories. How many looks can you create? Maybe there's a way to work in those unloved pieces that you hadn't considered before.

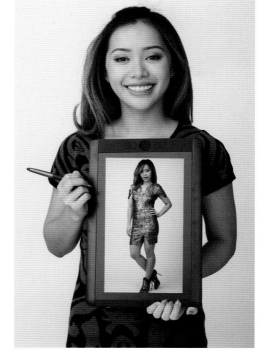

Write down each look. This will be a huge time-saver because you can refer to this list from now on whenever you need to get ready. You can even plan a whole week's worth of outfits in advance.

If you want to take this to the next level, photograph each look and start a private photo album you can reference. Or send the pictures to a friend with great taste and ask for his or her feedback.

THE BUILDING BLOCKS

There are four components to every good wardrobe: basics, classics, statement pieces, and investment pieces. When you find an item of clothing you'd like to buy, ask yourself which category it falls under. This will help you avoid impulse purchases you never wear. Some items might cross categories. Maybe you found a black blazer that's kind of expensive, but you know it will go with everything and you'll have it forever. That counts as a basic, a classic, and an investment piece!

The Basics

The basics are, well, basic items of clothing. Essential to a good wardrobe, these include any neutral-colored items you can build looks around. Basics are plain in construction and design. Unless you're in a punk rock band, a shredded pink T-shirt is not a basic. A flattering T-shirt in gray, black, or white is. Got it?

What do I consider must-have basics? A blazer, a pencil skirt, leggings, tights, pumps, a clutch, and a good everyday bag, all in black. And of course, jeans—the universal basic!

WEAR AND TEAR When shopping for basics, don't cheap out. I'm not saying you need to buy a $100 T-shirt, but you should calculate wear and tear. If you're going to wear a certain item a lot, it's okay to spend a little more if you can afford it and get a lot of quality in return. For that reason, I don't mind spending more on jackets, bags, shoes, and jeans. I wear them the most often and I need them to last! The things you wear most frequently shouldn't fall apart.

Often, you get what you pay for. Once when I was in the Los Angeles International Airport, my bag broke and busted right open. It was a cheap bag—and yes, I probably crammed too much stuff in it—but I realized right then and there that I needed to buy a better one. I knew I would have to spend more money, but at least I would get something sturdy and well made. Nothing makes you feel more disorganized and chaotic than the entire contents of your bag spilling on the floor at a busy airport!

The Classics

Classics are things you can wear at any age and in many situations. Think about some style icons from years past. What did they wear that would still look good today? The most classic items are a trench coat, a navy blazer, a crisp white shirt, a black-and-white-striped T-shirt, a black pencil skirt, and a black shift dress. These are pieces you can wear for years to come that can be dressed up or dressed down by pairing them with other items and accessories. Example? I can throw a chic black leather jacket over a black shift dress, add a fierce necklace, platform shoes, and a cool clutch, and I'm ready to go to a club. I can pair the same dress with a black blazer, sensible pumps, and a smart bag and head right to a job interview.

Investment Pieces

These are expensive items of clothing that you plan to wear frequently and/or own for a long time. An expensive trendy item is not an investment piece. Maybe you see a leather jacket that you love. You look at the price tag and you are ready to faint! But wait. How many times are you going to wear that leather jacket? It might be a good investment if you plan to own it for years and rock it a lot. You can amortize it. What does that mean? Say the jacket costs $500. If you plan to wear it twice a week for one year, that's roughly $5 per wearing. If you own it for a few years, you can get the cost down to $1 per wearing—or maybe less! It might be a better investment in the long run than a $50 item from a cheap store that you wear a few times and never again. It's fashion math, but it makes sense!

Be smart about any investment pieces. Look for things that will never go out of style. A designer name doesn't guarantee timelessness, but certain things do. A classic silhouette, meaning a slim trouser versus something low-rise and baggy, or a basic blazer versus one with the back cut out of it, for example. Certain colors are always classic, such as black, navy blue, and burgundy. Pastels and neon colors? Not so much. Tan and white are classics, but they get dirty fast. You don't want to spend a lot of money on a beautiful white coat only to have it stained within a few months.

Make sure any investment piece is well made. Take a good look at the construction. Are the buttons and seams sturdy? Is the piece lined? Is there some heft to the fabric? A high price doesn't always equal quality.

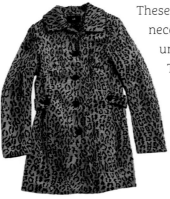

These are the items that catch people's eye. They're not trendy, necessarily, although they can be. They are pieces that are unique because of the designer, the color, or the silhouette. These pieces turn heads and make people say, "Wow. That's awesome." A statement piece can be a chic dress in a cool optical print, a fitted blazer in hot pink, or leopard-print coat. Anything that's not basic and neutral. Chances are, you won't wear your statement pieces frequently, but who knows? Maybe you like to make a statement every day!

DRESSING FOR YOUR BODY TYPE

Understanding your body is so important. It's truly the key to looking great. Once you know what flatters your shape, it's so much easier to put together looks you feel confident about. Where do you start? Well, look in the mirror. There are some basic body types that most people fit into: petite, tall, curvy, apple shaped, and inverted triangle. (You can cross categories as well. You might be petite and curvy, or a tall inverted triangle.)

Next, go online. Find some celebrities with a body type like yours—it's easy; just Google "curvy celebrities," "tall celebrities," "petite celebrities," etc. See whose style of dressing you like and what items of clothing look best on them. Is there anything in your wardrobe that's similar? Maybe there are pieces in your closet worth revisiting. Or maybe it's time to re-evaluate your wardrobe.

I've certainly made a lot of fashion mistakes over the years. I used to love buying jackets with really strong shoulders, but they didn't work on my petite five-foot frame. It turns out I need daintier things that don't overwhelm my body. I also liked midlength skirts, but the way they hit my calves made me look shorter. Same with ankle boots. Instead of flattering my legs, ankle boots make them look shorter because they cut off my leg at a certain point. It's all about fit and proportion. As for jeans, I've learned a higher waist is better than a low rise because it elongates my legs. And I'll never wear bell-bottoms again. A skinny leg is best for me.

Other things that work for me? Jumpers. They always look cute when you are petite. Same with short dresses and skirts or anything above the knee. They work proportionally. I also like nude shoes with bare legs because they give the illusion of length.

As you can see, it's about balancing and accentuating what you have, no matter what your shape or size. Below are a few tips for each body type. Don't consider these hard-and-fast rules, but rather suggestions. After all, there are a few celebrities who dress against body type and have made it their signature look. I'm sure you know the petite sisters who love wearing anything big and oversized, from dresses and coats to sunglasses. Then there is the famously curvy reality star who likes anything tight and trendy from major fashion designers. If you want to dress against type, it's okay. Just be brave and own it!

PETITE

- Match the color of your top and bottom. Monochromatic dressing (meaning one color from head to toe—say, black) is more lengthening than color-block dressing (where your top is one color and your pants or skirt are another color, say peach on top and navy on the bottom).
- Wear nude shoes with bare legs and black shoes with black tights for the illusion of length.
- Try a top with vertical stripes and pants with a tuxedo stripe.
- Go for a high-waisted pant or skirt rather than low rise.
- If you like heels, swap them for wedge sneakers when wearing something casual.

CURVY

- Wear form-fitting dresses and separates instead of oversize, shapeless clothing.
- Try pencil skirts that come right to the knee.
- Define your waist with an eye-catching belt.
- Go for solid colors instead of prints.
- Skip any tops with ruffles.

TALL

Most people want to look taller, so I'm not sure what advice to give if you're already tall! I know some girls don't like being taller than everyone around them, but embrace it. Go ahead and wear high heels. Be proud of what nature gave you and stand up straight! And be nice to your petite pals.

If you don't want to draw attention to your height, there are a few tricks you can try:

- Don't wear vertical stripes. Try a horizontal-striped shirt or dress instead.
- Go for color-block dressing.
- Wear flats. They look chic for daytime or even black tie.

APPLE

- Look for V-neck tops.
- Straight-legged pants are a better choice than leggings.
- Try wrap dresses and wrap blouses to help you fake a waistline.
- Avoid high necklines and A-line dresses.
- Color-block your clothes instead of wearing all one color.

INVERTED TRIANGLE

- Go for soft-shouldered tops and jackets to de-emphasize your shoulders.
- Avoid any major shoulder-pad action.
- Choose items that accentuate your waistline, like nipped-in blazers and cool belts.
- Look for fuller skirts to balance your top and bottom.
- Skip shirts with horizontal stripes.

DRESSING FOR DIFFERENT OCCASIONS

Sometimes it's hard to know what to wear for a specific occasion. You don't want to be too dressed up; at the same time, you don't want to look too casual. If you're unclear on the right thing to wear, it's always better to overdress than underdress. When you are underdressed, it can signal that you don't care. Being overdressed shows that you put some effort and thought into it. But use your common sense. You wouldn't wear a ball gown to a baseball game—unless you're trying to make a major statement!

Here are some ideas for what to wear for certain situations.

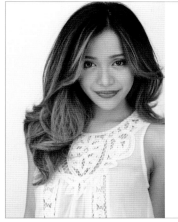

FIRST DATE

The most important thing is looking like your true self. Don't dress like a different person on a first date. Otherwise, when do you plan to reveal the real you? On the third date? Fourth date? Never?

Definitely don't dress like you're heading to a night-club—unless that's where the first date is! I would go with something pretty and pulled together.

WEDDING

You should always look nice at a wedding. A dress or a suit is the only appropriate attire. Anything ripped or torn is not respectful to those getting married. Whatever you do, don't wear white! The bride has the exclusive right to that color on her wedding day.

FUNERAL

Again, it's all about respect. A funeral or memorial service is about remembering the person we've lost, so don't ever dress in a showy or sloppy manner. In most countries, it's appropriate to wear dark colors, such as black or navy. I think other colors are okay, as long as they aren't bold or bright, such as red, bright pink, or yellow.

In certain Asian cultures, you wear white to a funeral.

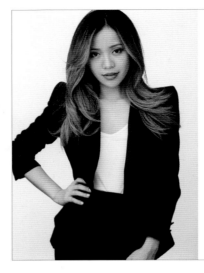

JOB INTERVIEW
Your outfit can make or break your chances of getting a job. I talk about this extensively later on. Before your interview, do a little homework and find out what people wear at the workplace. Wear something similar to the interview, or go a little dressier. For example, if the employees wear jeans, hoodies, and sneakers, wear a nice pair of jeans and a T-shirt with a blazer and a pair of boots or flats. You can wear the hoodie when you get the actual job! This is your chance to make a good impression.

WORK

This requires an entire section, so let's go!

WORK WEAR

I find that workplaces fall into two categories. You have the places where people can wear what they like and individuality is okay. And at other places, employees wear a "uniform." By that I mean a certain look that all the employees tend to adopt. If you don't wear the uniform, you won't fit in and you might not be taken seriously. If you hate the uniform, you are probably in the wrong job.

Let's take a look at the "uniform" for a few different professions.

TECH START-UP EMPLOYEE

These modern workplaces seemingly have the most lenient of dress codes, yet uniforms are prized here as well. It might be hard to view these outfits as uniforms because they are so casual, but don't let that fool you. A uniform is a uniform! Remember how Steve Jobs used to dress when he was running Apple? Jeans, black turtleneck, New Balance sneakers? He was one of the most powerful and successful men in the world, but he stuck to a very specific, very casual look. Same with Facebook founder Mark Zuckerberg in his gray T-shirt, hoodie, and jeans. It's about dressing like a regular person but signaling that you're above fashion with your relentless consistency.

For the most part, dressing in the tech world is about comfort. Days are long at a start-up and you spend a lot of time at your desk. The only time you really think about your clothes is when you meet with clients or investors. Those are the occasions when you want to make a good impression, so ditch the flip-flops and the wrinkled T-shirt.

Yes

- Denim
- Sneakers or flip-flops
- Hoodies
- T-shirts
- Headphones

No-no

- Smelly, wrinkled clothes. There's not much time for laundry when you're at a start-up. You pretty much roll out of bed every day and head straight to work. But think of your colleagues! Find a clean T-shirt.
- Bare feet. I've seen programmers walk around the Google offices with no shoes on, but I wouldn't recommend it.

TRADITIONAL/CORPORATE EMPLOYEE

We're talking about jobs in finance and law. Your workplace might even have written guidelines about what you can wear. Anything crazy or trendy is definitely out of the question. Wardrobe wise, the idea is to blend in. You don't want to stand out; you are part of a team. It's the work—or the client—that matters. But that doesn't mean you need to dress in a completely boring or unisex way. Look for beautifully cut clothes that are made out of nice fabrics. Also, pay attention to your hair and makeup. When your clothes are conservative, you don't want to disappear completely.

Yes

- Neutral colors
- Modest silhouettes
- Simple accessories
- A stylish computer bag
- Sensible shoes

No-no

- Shoes that make noise when you walk
- Jewelry that clinks and clacks
- Short skirts or dresses
- Exposed cleavage
- Bright colors

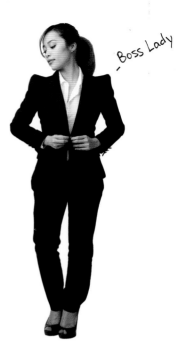

— Boss Lady

TEACHER

Dress how you want the kids to see you. I think it's best when teachers dress modestly and in a timeless, classic way. You never want to look too casual or like you care too much about fashion. At the same time, you don't want to look too severe, like you work at a financial institution. You might send the message that you aren't approachable.

Yes

- Comfortable shoes (you'll be standing a lot!)
- Comfortable clothes
- Blackboard-compatible clothing! You don't want to reveal any body parts when you reach to write at the top of the chalkboard. Make sure your tops come well below the waist of your pants or skirts.
- Jewel tones
- Simple jewelry

No-no

- Miniskirts
- Low-cut blouses
- Casual denim (torn, baggy, etc.)
- Sweatpants
- High heels

A+

FASHION

People who work in fashion have to be very conscious of how they dress. Stay on top of the trends. If you don't care about how you dress, don't go into this industry. Fashion professionals definitely care how you look. It's just the way it is. Figure out what the "voice" is where you work and make sure your clothing matches. By "voice," I mean the tone or overall vibe of the place. Is it downtown chic, uptown sophisticated, super fashion-forward?

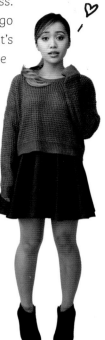

Yes
- The color black
- Designer clothing
- Trends in moderation
- A statement item (cool shoes, necklace, hat, etc.)

No-no
- Knockoffs or anything counterfeit
- Cheap trendy items
- Preppy, conservative looks
- Boot-cut jeans

ARTIST

This is probably the one profession where you can wear whatever you want. It's all about image. If you're an artist, you're a bit like a character in a story. What is that story? What do you want to tell the world? Make sure your look relates to your vision. There are no yeses or no-nos because anything goes.

STREET-STYLE STAR

You need a lot of connections and a lot of style for this rare job. You might have better luck running for president or getting drafted into the NBA! If it's your dream, go for it. The wardrobe is certainly killer, but you need to make sure some of your best friends are fashion designers. After all, you need to borrow clothes the second they come off the runway. Once the clothes are in stores, you don't touch them.

Yes

- Fearless mixing of prints and patterns
- The crazier the shoe, the better
- Clutches
- Bold colors
- Sunglasses
- Camera-ready hair and makeup

No-no

- Last season's clothes
- Anything a celebrity already wore
- All black
- Seasonally appropriate gear (Snow boots? A coat? C'mon! You'd never cover up your outfit.)

FASHION STYLISTS/MAKEUP ARTISTS/ HAIRSTYLISTS

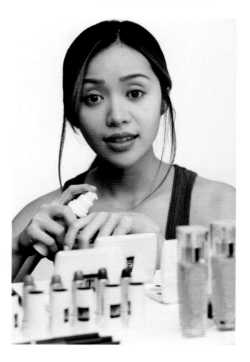

When it comes to these professions, how you look depends on where you live. The West Coast is definitely in one camp, and the East Coast and Europe are in another. On the West Coast, it's all about your look. L.A. is a celebrity world, so that means it's okay if you dress like one too. You want people to say, "Wow, you must be really good because you look the part." In L.A., if you're a fashion stylist, your look reflects your work. If your signature style is romantic, you dress romantic. Edgy, you dress edgy. Makeup artists and hairdressers dress uniquely as well and put a lot of their personality into it.

In New York, it's about your work and not caring how you look. In Europe, it's more about minimalism. You might have a hard time believing this, but a lot of top female makeup artists I know don't wear makeup! I didn't believe that at first either, but it's true. If they wear any, it's the no-makeup makeup look—a bit of concealer to cover any dark circles, a hint of blush for some color, a tinted lip balm, maybe a bit of mascara.

Yes
- Anything black
- Chic sneakers
- Jeans
- Dirty hair
- No makeup
- High/low (designer items mixed with chain-store bargains)

No-no
- Trendy clothing
- Anything fancy or fussy
- Clothes you can't move around in

MODESTY

Some people think if you have it, you should rock it, but I'm in favor of dressing modestly, especially at work. There's something mysterious and elegant about modesty. When in doubt, cover up a little bit. Keep it classy and don't go crazy with the cleavage. As for short shorts, please don't. Your butt cheeks should never hang below the fabric. Even if you have the best butt in the world, it's not a good look.

REPEAT IT!

Don't ever be afraid to repeat an outfit. The chicest women in the world wear the same clothes over and over—princesses, editors in chief, first ladies, they all do it. Style has nothing to do with owning tons of the latest stuff and wearing a new outfit every day.

You should never feel like you need to keep up with the Joneses, as the expression goes. Ten years from now, no one will care about the Joneses. It's your life that you're living, so don't focus on anyone else but you. This is your story. Focus on you!

HOW TO ACCESSORIZE

When it comes to accessorizing my look, I keep it simple. To be honest, I don't go all-out on accessories because I go all-out on makeup. I generally wear a bracelet and a ring, and if I'm leaving the house, I always have a bag, of course, and sunglasses. I prefer aviators. I'm not a fan of big bug sunglasses because they don't work for my face size and shape.

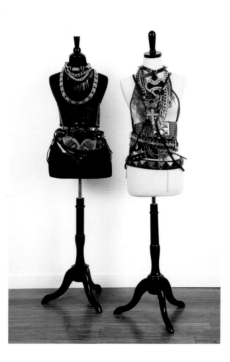

Accessories can be your best friend and really help stretch your wardrobe. With the right items, you can make a basic dress or top and skirt look pretty, punky, sexy, or conservative.

Everyone thinks accessories are one size fits all, but you do need to take body shape into account. I'd love to wear an armful of bangles and do the whole arm-candy thing, but it would make my arms look shorter than they already are. Same with big necklaces, earrings, scarves, belts, and handbags. I love a big bag, but I disappear if I'm wearing or carrying anything oversize. You also want to take the shape of the accessory into consideration. Think about the difference between a big colorful scarf and a thin, long black one. Same as a purse. Something square and colorful will draw attention to itself and look blocky, while something more streamlined, say a classic soft-sided rectangular purse on a chain, could help elongate you.

GLASSES

My eyesight isn't perfect, so I need to wear glasses sometimes. Because of the way my nose is shaped, many glasses slip right off. I really need to shop around to find a pair that fits my face. If you wear glasses, keep your face shape in mind when selecting a pair. You want to play up the shape, not work against it. I know thick frames are really in style right now, but personally, I prefer a thinner frame with a decorative element, like a bit of leopard or color on the sides.

ROUND If your face is round, you probably have full cheeks and a soft chin line and forehead.

To help add definition to your face, look for glasses with strong angular shapes or rectangular frames. This will give the illusion of a longer face shape. Rectangular glasses can also help widen the eyes. Avoid circular glasses, like something Harry Potter would rock. General rule of thumb: Pick out a frame shape that is the opposite of your face shape.

SQUARE If you have a strong jaw and broad forehead, then you're a square . . . your face shape, not your personality! Your face shape is very high-fashion.

A gorgeous strong face shape like yours works well with glasses that are softer and rounder. Look for glasses that sit high on the nose. This will lengthen the face. Try to find a frame with a heavier top line that brings attention back to the center of your face instead of your jawline. Your frames should soften your strong features, not accentuate them. It's all about bringing balance to your face, so that means avoiding overly boxy, narrow frames.

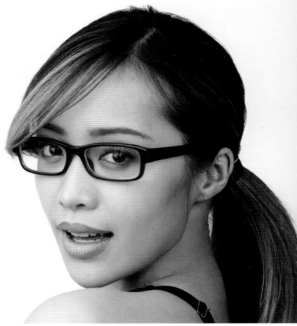

DIAMOND If you have a narrow forehead and jawline, you are a diamond.

You can play up your delicate features with fun cat-eye and oval shapes. Glasses that sweep up will help emphasize your cheekbones. Also, decoration on the top of the frames will help add width to your brows. Avoid boxy, straight-across frames that might accentuate the width of your cheeks. Keep it delicate and sassy.

OBLONG If your face is an oval, you have the oblong face shape.

Try oversized glasses, especially those that are wider than your face. Decorative bold rims will look great on you.

HOW TO WEAR HEELS

The first time you wear high heels can be awkward. After all, you're walking on your tippy-toes. If you're a newbie, try kitten heels first and work your way up. (A kitten heel is a thin heel that is an inch and a half in length or shorter.) If you do fall or stumble, don't be embarrassed. I fell so many times when I was learning to walk in heels! Get right back up and laugh it off.

When shopping for heels, remember that the thicker the heel, the more balance it provides. If you plan to walk in these shoes, or hop on the bus or subway, keep that in mind. Also, make sure the shoes fit well. High heels are chic, but blisters and a foot full of Band-Aids are not!

One last word of advice—if you are wearing heels and going up or down stairs, use the handrail! Stairs and heels aren't the best mix. I know girls who have taken bad spills on stairs, so don't let that happen to you.

SMART SHOPPING

Even though I can afford more things today than when I was younger, I always ask myself, "Do I really need this?" I was shopping online recently because I had to find a dress for a movie premiere. I found a beautiful one, but it cost a fortune. I told myself, "If I'm going to spend this much money, I need to wear it a million times." So I looked around for something else and even found a coupon I could use. I don't care how rich or poor you are; if you can find a good deal, that's the best thing. Be a smart, savvy shopper. It's always good to save money.

VINTAGE SHOPPING

If you don't have a lot of money or you want to look unique, shopping in thrift stores or vintage boutiques is the way to go. Look at how many celebrities, models, and style icons love vintage clothing. There's something special about wearing a piece with history to it.

I love shopping at flea markets and vintage boutiques because you can find really beautiful things that are one of a kind. You certainly won't bump into anyone wearing the same outfit when you scored it at a secondhand shop! When I was at art school in Sarasota, shopping at the local Goodwill was like going on a treasure hunt. A lot of wealthy retired people live in that town and would donate their things. You could find Chanel jackets and Louis Vuitton bags for a fraction of what they would cost in a boutique. However, it does take patience and a good eye to make a great score.

How do you develop a good eye? For one thing, study fashion magazines or look at fashion shows online. Figure out what makes something classic or super-of-the-moment trendy. See what respected celebrities wear on the red carpet and what does and doesn't work for them. Also, develop an understanding of what makes an item well made. We talked about this earlier. Does the fabric have a little weight to it? Do the buttons look and feel sturdy? Are they sewn on well? How are the seams and the stitching? Does the garment have a lining? Next time you are in a clothing store, pick up an item and really look at it. Turn it inside out and see what the construction is like. You'll be surprised how much you learn just by looking, touching, and comparing.

ONLINE SHOPPING

Shopping for clothes online can get you into trouble. It's easy and it's fun, but someone has to pay for those purchases! Be careful of impulse shopping. If you buy something that doesn't fit or that you regret, return it promptly. It's okay to make a shopping mistake, but make sure you get your money back. Don't punish your bank account.

HOW TO CARE FOR YOUR CLOTHES AND SHOES

You should always take good care of your things. Whether expensive or inexpensive, clothing and shoes last longer when they're treated with a little love.

HAND-WASHING HOW-TO

When it comes to washing your clothing, make sure to read the label and understand the material. Some things can go into the washing machine, other things need to be dry-cleaned or hand-washed. Not sure how to hand-wash your things? I use a big plastic bowl and fill it with warm water (cold water if the item is dark) and a bit of OxiClean. I put the item in the bowl and let it soak for a little while. If there is a stain, I use the same side of the material and rub the stain gently with the clean side, then rinse it well. Next, I put the item on a towel and reshape it. Leave it for at least an hour. This way the towel absorbs a lot of the moisture. (Don't do this on a wooden floor! You could warp your floors.)

For the final step, I hang the item and let it air-dry. If you skip the towel step, your clothes will drip water everywhere when you hang them.

SHOE CARE

Back in the days when I was a broke college student, I had one nice pair of shoes. I took meticulous care of them because they were my only option. I made sure to polish and buff them regularly, especially when they got scuffed. There are all kinds of shoe polish you can use to make your shoes look new. For dark shoes, there is cream or liquid polish. If you have white shoes, you can use those Mr. Clean Magic Erasers to buff off any marks and make them as good as new. For suede shoes, use a white or pink eraser to remove any kind of salt or sweat stains. If you wear down the heels or soles of your shoes, or break a heel, take them to a local shoe-repair shop. Shoes can last for years if you take care of them.

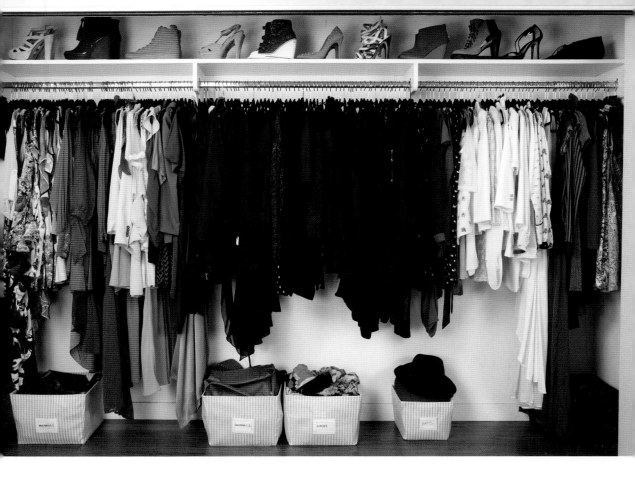

ORGANIZE YOUR CLOTHES

I store my clothes according to the seasons. In Los Angeles, the seasons don't differ that much. In New York, however, the weather can change from day to day. It might be ninety degrees and sunny one day, thirty-five with driving rain the next. Or snow! So you need to be prepared. My main closet has the items I need for the current season; everything else goes into storage. It's all about maximizing square footage and being efficient. I know some girls like having a big crazy wardrobe where you can go in and just grab whatever. But I don't. I don't need to see every single thing I own.

I'm very specific about how I organize my closet. The order goes from tops to bottoms, with each category getting its own section: jackets, blouses, leggings, skirts, etc. Each section is color-coordinated. This way I can go in and find what I need without wasting any time. When I

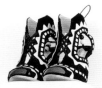

SHOE STORAGE

If you spend a lot of money on shoes, you don't want to hide them away. I use a system of big stacking storage cubes, which makes it easy to see everything and decide what I want to wear that day. I don't like regular shoe racks where you have to bend down and grab everything.

remove an article of clothing, I always put the empty hanger back so I can see exactly where the item needs to go when I'm finished wearing it. I'm not crazy specific about the type of hanger, although I do like those thin velour hangers. Clothes don't slip off them.

As for my accessories, I organize them on a little tree made for that purpose. If you have a lot of bracelets, rings, necklaces, and other things to organize, you can use one of those hanging bags with multiple clear compartments. You see everything at a glance, and it's great for travel. Or get creative and use a pegboard to display everything.

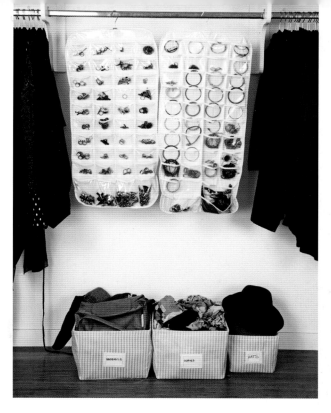

THE FINAL WORD ON FASHION

Do not let material things define who you are. The true you is reflected by your intelligence, your character, your personality, and your actions. These are things that money can't buy and that never go out of fashion.

Earlier in this book, I talked about trying on different outfits and personalities in high school as a way to fit in. I don't regret those attempts at figuring out who the real me was. I think we all go through versions of that as we try to identify our true selves and what is meaningful to us.

Nothing's more stylish than knowing who you are. Be a woman of substance, not a woman of stuff.

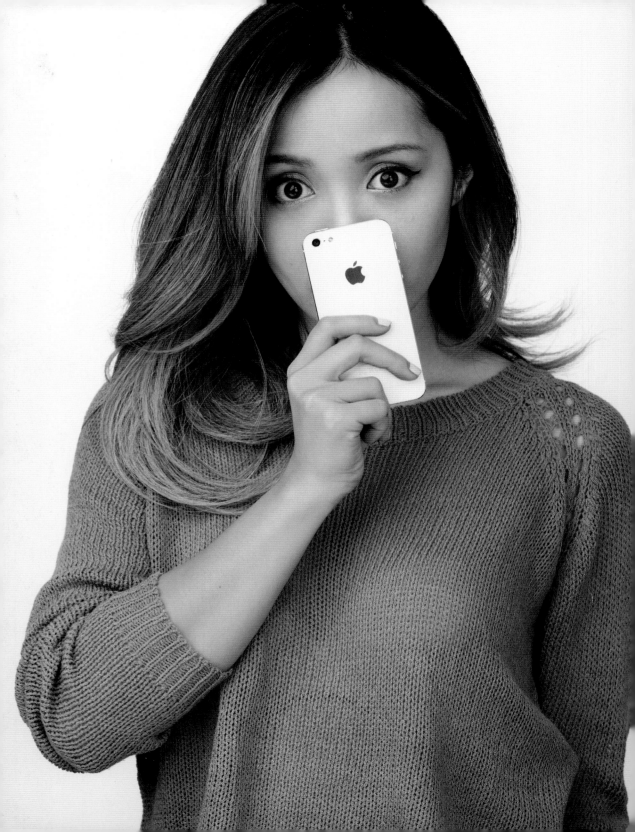

DIGITAL DOS AND DON'TS

No matter what anyone says, it's not easy navigating the digital space. My whole life revolves around the digital space, and I still find it tricky! The rules of engagement change all the time, the technology evolves constantly, and we're left holding these gadgets or staring at our computers, wondering what to do, how to do it, and why.

The Internet has been around for decades, but every day we encounter online situations that require a new set of thinking and behavior. It's kind of dizzying, isn't it? As soon as we master one thing, something better, cooler, and newer comes along. The immediacy of digital has changed our lives for the better, but it is a blessing and a curse. In this chapter, I'm going to share everything I've learned about dealing with the digital world—the ethics, the etiquette, the best practices. If you approach your digital life in a smart, strategic way, trust me—you'll have less to worry about and more time to enjoy the benefits!

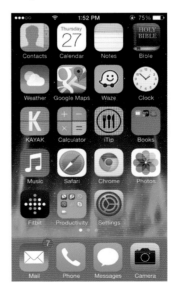

THE ART OF TEXTING

Texting is such a quick, easy way to communicate. Type out a few words and hit send. Many people barely talk on the phone or leave voice mail messages anymore because texting is so convenient. But like all forms of written communication, there is so much potential for misunderstanding.

Let's go over a few ground rules.

REPLY PROMPTLY

Got a message? A few hours ago? Yesterday? What are you waiting for? I'm not saying drop everything and respond, but most messages should be returned within a reasonable amount of time. If not, the person who sent the message is going to wonder how much you care. For example, let's say your friend sends you a text. You don't respond, but he or she can see that you did have time to update your Facebook status and post a new picture on Instagram. That might be hurtful. Try to respond to texts within an hour of their being sent. However, if you're at work, on a date, or doing something else that requires your time and attention, it can wait.

Of course, there are exceptions to the rule. Maybe someone sent you a text that requires a thoughtful response. In that case, definitely take your time to mull over what you are going to say. Or perhaps you are sending a message by deliberately delaying your response. If you wait a day or so, that message will be loud and clear.

Can you ignore a text message? Of course! But you will definitely be communicating that you are mad or indifferent. You can always pretend you didn't get the text, but that white lie is hard to believe these days! It's easier to believe that you simply didn't see a text and it got lost among the others. Of course, if the sender is a stranger or someone you barely know, you're under no obligation to respond.

TEXTING DOS AND DON'TS

Don't send a novel. If your text requires a lot of words to get your point across, move it to e-mail.

Hey, I wasn't sure if you got my message but I think we should definitely meet sometime this week to go over our project. I have so many great ideas I'd like to run by you. I was thinking that we could start out with an opening Power Point presentation and then incorporate an activity. Maybe we can even end with a prize! If you have time now let me know what you think. If not we can talk in class tomorrow.

Don't write in all caps. It's considered THE EQUIVALENT OF YELLING. (See?) If you are trying to make a point loudly, that's fine. But if not, use the upper and lower cases properly.

> Hey, I'm really sorry, but I don't think that I'll be able to make it to the event tonight.

OK. WHY NOT? ← whoa there

> Sorry...didn't mean to offend you. My sister surprised me and came into town a day early.

Oh, no worries. I'll see you next week.

Don't respond to a long, important, or meaningful text message with "K." It can come off as insulting. Put a little more effort into it or the person on the other end will take it the wrong way. "K" is only okay if you need to end the conversation quickly. Adding a smiling face is helpful: "K :)"

> Hey, I heard that you are coming to town this weekend! We should definitely catch up. Maybe we can get dinner. It would be great to see you. Let me know if you're free!

K

↖ not cool

Don't end your text messages with "..." unless you're unsure of something or you want to continue the conversation. (Those three dots, by the way, are called ellipses.) It implies that you might have more to say or you are discontent with something. For example, "Hey, I can't stop by today." "Oh, okay..." That is an invitation to say, "What's wrong?" Those three little dots are just as dramatic as a cliffhanger. Use them wisely.

> Want to go out tonight? We were thinking of having a girls' night downtown!

Yeah...

← don't leave them hanging!

> Well, we're leaving at 8 so tell me if you want to go before then.

Sure...

Do use emoticons or abbreviations appropriately. They're fun and silly, so enjoy them. Go ahead and use ILY, IRLY, and OMG with your friends. But your boss or landlord or anyone who's not your BFF? No.

> Hi____, this is ____ from work. Could you please sign the package that is coming in tomorrow?

OMG thank you for reminding me!
I will totally stay in the front office
to sign for it. C u l8r! ☺

Don't sext. Do we even need to talk about this? I've seen too many guys and girls share racy texts they received with others. Nothing is private, even though you think it might be.

Don't fight via text. It's better to pick up the phone and have it out. Arguing through text messages achieves nothing but a lot of bitter back-and-forth.

Don't end a relationship via text message. (Or via Facebook!) The only excuse for not doing this in person or over the phone is if the person is dangerous and might react violently. Someone broke up with me via text, and let me tell you, I have no respect for that guy. It's disrespectful to end something this way.

> Hey, I know we've just started dating, but I don't think that this is working out. I'm sorry.

Are you breaking up with me?!?!

> Yeah, I just can't do this anymore.

ARE YOU KIDDING ME?? Over text? Really? ← *really?*

Don't text while impaired. And don't let friends do that either. Actually, don't do any social media of any kind while impaired. It's a recipe for disaster!

Don't text while driving. This is the most important thing I'm going to tell you in this chapter. It only takes a second to get into an accident. If you are a passenger and the driver starts texting, insist that he or she stop. Offer to send the text for the driver. There's no reason to text while driving. Our parents didn't drive around and text—the message can wait until you park the car.

ADDICTED TO POSTING?

How often do you update your favorite social media platforms? Weekly? Once a day? Hourly? If you update multiple times a day, it might be too much. It's one thing to answer people on Twitter and have a back-and-forth conversation, but to post ten Instagram photos a day? Or half a dozen Facebook status updates? That just not polite or a good use of your time. You are clogging up your friends' and followers' feeds. You need to edit. Quality over quantity. Rein yourself in and decide what the most essential message, photo, or update is. Otherwise, you might find that people stop following you or unfriend you.

There are a few exceptions. Amazing meals, trips, and conferences? Things like that get a pass. Of course I'd love to see your pictures if you're covering Paris Fashion Week for work. But let's not upload blurry pictures of a model walking down a runway. It's a waste of space on your friends' feeds. Are you on safari in Africa, surrounded by lions and elephants? Yes, post away (if you have a connection, that is!). Are you a professional photographer? You get a pass too. But again, remember to edit yourself.

Everyone's life is amazing, so give others a chance!

What if you're addicted to posting? That is definitely a problem. You need to ask yourself why you crave the attention and the validation it brings. Are you a social (media) butterfly who lives for the thumbs-up? Your life shouldn't be about what other people think. It's about what you think!

You might need a digital detox, which I talk about later in this chapter.

You don't need to go cold turkey, but you should give yourself limits. Try to reduce the time you spend posting each day until you are down to a reasonable number of posts. Your actual life could be passing you by if you spend too much time on your virtual life. One post per day per platform is plenty, unless it's a special day. One exception is Twitter. If you're having a conversation with someone, it's fine to tweet back and forth a few times.

POSTING DOS AND DON'TS

Do share major moments with your friends and followers.

Don't hog the news feed. People will roll their eyes and scroll past your updates if you post too much.

Don't let updates become an obsession. It's unhealthy.

THE DANGER OF OVERSHARING

We just talked about posting too much, which is a form of oversharing. But there's a more dangerous form of oversharing, and that's letting the world know too much of your business. The success of social media is built on this ongoing cycle of sharing. Some people share because it validates them; some because they want to share experiences with the world and have others experience them too.

But when it comes to your private life, you need to be very careful what you reveal. If you want to share your most intimate details, that's a decision you have to make. However, I think it's important to keep your private life sacred. Whatever you put in the online world is there *forever.* You can never take it back. Sure, you can delete it, but remember that anyone can take a screenshot and share it widely.

Maybe you and your friends have a crazy night. All of it is captured on your iPhone and you decide to put a few pictures on your Facebook page. What's the harm? Your parents aren't on Facebook. You're not Facebook friends with your boss.

Well, other people can see it. And it turns out that employers and human resources departments look at the social media activity of potential job candidates. It's not illegal to do so. If you are as qualified as another candidate, your social media content could be the difference between getting the job or not getting the job.

Before you show the world your wild side, or private side, or gross, silly side, think about it: If someone sees this five years from now, what will they think? As boring as it sounds, I do believe you need to censor yourself. It's no different from when you are speaking. You can't just blurt out the first thing that comes to mind. You think before you speak, and you need to think before you post. I have a personal test that I run everything through. I ask myself if I would want the daughter I hope to have one day to see this when she is older. If not, I don't post it.

Sometimes I look at the most popular pictures on Instagram to see what's trending, and I'm shocked. So many young girls post the raunchiest photos. It's obvious they're only teenagers and I can't help but wonder what they are doing. Are they desperate for approval or validation? Maybe, but it's the wrong kind of validation, from the wrong kind of people.

It's not just social media, by the way. Maybe you have a sexy photo of yourself that you want to text to your boyfriend or girlfriend, or someone you're interested in. Unless you want the world to see it, don't do it! So many things can happen. The recipient can forward the picture to anyone. (That happened to a friend of mine on Snapchat, where things like that aren't supposed to occur. The guy she was communicating with took a screenshot of the intimate picture she sent him.) His or her phone can get stolen. Someone can hack into his or her account. You can accidentally send it to the wrong person. It happens to celebrities, it's ruined the careers of politicians, and it's devastated the lives of everyday people. These are extreme instances, of course. It might seem incredibly innocent in the moment, but I want you to think before you hit send or post or tweet.

A quick note about workplace oversharing! It's not just raunchy photos that can ruin your career prospects. Some people completely overshare about work business. You should never post any kind of grievance you might have with your boss, your colleagues, or your customers. They might not "follow" you or be "friends" with you on social media, but it doesn't mean they can't see what you post. Keep work business private. Your boss might be mean, your coworkers might not be the smartest people, and maybe your customers are rude, but you could lose your job if you share those thoughts and feelings with the world. It's not worth it. If your job is that terrible, look for a new one.

OVERSHARING DOS AND DON'TS

Oversharing is always a don't.

Do consider your overall online image.

Do think about your future before posting certain comments, photos, or status updates.

Don't post or share anything that could ruin your reputation.

Don't gripe about your job, boss, or coworkers online.

ONLINE ROMANCE

More and more couples meet online today, through either dating websites or social media. There used to be some stigma attached to this, but these days it's a totally normal way to meet your boyfriend or girlfriend. Really: It's perfectly fine. I've read that one-third of all married couples meet online. That's a significant number, and it's growing!

It's nice to have a choice today. You can meet someone the old-fashioned way, or you can take matters into your own hands and be a bit more specific about the kind of person you'd like to meet. Is height important? Or religion or education level? You can be as particular as you like. There are so many dating sites you can join. You just need to find the one that's right for you.

Once you decide to explore online dating, there are a few rules you should follow. It's so easy to be fooled in the online world. Remember that story about the college football player with the fake girlfriend? Sadly, there are devious types out there looking to take advantage of people, so you have to be on alert. I'm not saying you need to be suspicious of everyone, but you do need to be a detective of sorts.

That goes both ways! If you're putting together your profile for an online dating site, keep it factual. Are you really a certain height, weight, or age? Do you really have that level of education? Don't exaggerate the truth.

So, let's start at the beginning. You meet someone online and you start talking. You kind of like this person. You talk some more, you're getting to know each other. You make plans to meet. Stop right there. What do you know about this person? Research the heck out of them. The Internet has given you the tools to be smart about the choices you make, whether it's what car to buy, what restaurant to visit, or what movie to watch. It's no different when we're talking about a relationship. Do not feel bad about doing this. Why would you do more research about a *Star Trek* movie or a car than someone you might be with for the rest of your life?

Before I dated anyone, you'd better believe I researched everything—his name, his residence, his employment. I even looked at websites that list local predators. I rolled up my sleeves and acted as my own private investigator.

Be super smart. Don't suspend your judgment just because you really like someone. It's good to be careful and guarded in the beginning, maybe even a little suspicious. Now, that said, you can't always be looking for something bad. At some point, your partner deserves the benefit of the doubt. If your general nature is suspicious, you might have a hard time with online dating. You'd be better off dating someone in your neighborhood or someone who knows your group of friends—basically, someone who can be validated by another person.

If the object of your affection is legitimate, congratulations! I hope you two have a long, healthy relationship.

Ultimately, for all relationships to work, you need three things:

Communication

Honesty

Respect

ONLINE DATING DOS AND DON'TS

Don't lie about who you are. It's a terrible way to start a relationship. Besides, you want someone who loves you for you.

Don't suspend your judgment. Trust your instincts. If something doesn't seem right, it's probably not.

Do your homework! You don't need a private detective to check someone out. The Internet makes it easy to do it yourself.

Do trust the other person . . . once you've checked him or her out.

Don't be afraid to fall in love.

PUT YOUR DEVICES AWAY

When you are spending time with others, give them your full attention. Nothing is sadder than a group of people fixated on their devices rather than one another.

DEVICE DOS AND DON'TS

Do put away your device at the start of a meal.

Don't take out your device at inappropriate times. You know what I'm talking about.

Don't walk down the sidewalk or cross the street while looking at your device. I know of people who've fallen into potholes or gotten hit by cars! Be aware of your surroundings.

PROFESSIONAL COMMUNICATIONS

When you are e-mailing for work, school, or some other serious purposes, be careful about the tone you use. If you are communicating with someone senior to you, you always want to convey a sense of professionalism.

For example:

hey, want some starbucks? I'm sending the intern.

Or

Good morning, Michelle. The intern is going to Starbucks to pick up some coffee for the meeting. Would you like her to get you something?

Best,
Wendy

Can you see the difference?

PROFESSIONAL COMMUNICATION DOS AND DON'TS

Do use proper names.

Do sign off with a closing and your name.

Don't use informal words like *hey* or terms like *K*.

Do check for spelling and grammar mistakes before hitting send.

Do convey a professional tone with colleagues and anyone senior to you.

Don't be too casual.

Do save personal thoughts for your personal e-mail, preferably sent from your home computer.

ONLINE ARGUMENTS

Fighting online is such a waste of time and never ends well for anyone. Whether you're at fault or the other person is totally wrong, you look equally bad. If you're the one being confrontational, you need to ask yourself why. What do you think you'll gain by fighting publicly?

Another problem with fighting online is that it creates a permanent record. You can't take things back. If you're going to say something, make sure you really mean it. It's so easy for your words to get twisted and for the actual meaning to get lost. I've said things I didn't mean and wished I could take them back, but I can't. I learned the hard way.

If you can walk away from an online fight, you are the stronger person. Ignoring is the weapon of choice. No one gets hurt.

Sometimes you just need perspective. Turn off your computer or put your device away and do something else. Come back twenty minutes later and see if you still feel the same way. When you feel passionate about something, you're not always thinking clearly. You are speaking from your heart, not your brain. That's not the worst thing, but you do need to consider the ramifications if your emotions get the best of you.

FIGHTING DOS AND DON'TS

Don't fight online. It's that simple.

Do take it offline. Sometimes a disagreement is legitimate, but that doesn't mean you need to share it with the world. Discuss your differences via e-mail, over the phone, or in person.

Do realize that anything on social media leaves a permanent record. You can go back and delete something, but anyone can take a screenshot.

Do sleep on it! It's best not to do things impulsively, and maybe rest will give you some needed perspective.

BE A GOOD DIGITAL BUDDY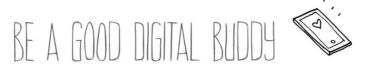

I mentioned this a little bit already, but when it comes to some digital issues, you need to be a good friend. Your pals won't always exercise the best judgment, so don't be afraid to speak up and save them from potential embarrassment or danger.

Say your friend wants to drive to her ex-boyfriend's house and sit outside in her car. You would stop her from doing that, wouldn't you? It's no different when it comes to your friend sending him a text, tagging him in an Instagram picture, or stalking his Facebook page.

Sometimes it's as easy as grabbing her phone and talking some sense into her. If you happen to see something your friend posted online that is inappropriate, don't be afraid to suggest he or she take it down. Your friend might appreciate the gesture. After all, you're looking out for his or her best interest.

DIGITAL BUDDY DOS AND DON'TS

Do speak up if your friend is about to send a text or post something on social media that he or she will regret.

Don't let your friends text and drive. Offer to send the text for them.

Don't ever snatch a phone away from a driver. In trying to prevent an accident, you could cause one. Just calmly tell your friend you don't want to be in the car if he or she is going to text and could they please pull over, stop the car, and finish the text.

Don't let your friends drink and post or text. It might seem funny, but everyone will regret it the next day.

Do alert a friend if something he or she posted is inappropriate. In the heat of the moment, he or she might not realize it wasn't a good idea.

WE ALL MAKE MISTAKES

Everyone will do something stupid online at least once in his or her life. I certainly have! So what do you do when that happens? Your only choice is to take responsibility and move on. Just come out and say, "Yeah, it was stupid. I wasn't thinking." Depending on the situation, you might want to add that you're a changed person now.

And yes, you can delete something if you regret posting it. Go ahead. But as I've warned a few times, anyone could take a screenshot. If you get called out for deleting something, you can admit to that too. "I realized it was [dumb/inappropriate/silly], so I took it down."

It can be very powerful to own up to your actions. If you're always hiding and running away from taking responsibility, people will use it against you. No one can do that if you turn your weakness or mistake around and use it as a shield. Then they have no ammunition. When people see your acknowledgment, they often move on.

MISTAKE DOS AND DON'TS

Do admit to your mistakes.

Do move on once you've owned up to your actions and/or apologized. The more you dwell on it, the more it continues to exist.

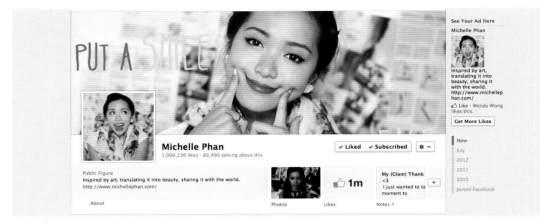

Michelle Phan
1,000,136 likes · 82,490 talking about this

✓ Liked   ✓ Subscribed   ⚙ ▾

Now
July
2012
2011
2010
Joined Facebook

Public Figure
Inspired by art, translating it into beauty, sharing it with the world.
http://www.michellephan.com/

👍 **1m**

My (Glam) Thank
<3
I just wanted to ta
moment to

About   Photos   Likes   Notes 4

WHAT IS YOUR ONLINE PERSONA?

Do you ever stop and think about the persona you project online? What does that mean exactly? Well, let's look at it in Hollywood terms. Let's say you are Actress A, who always does horror movies, poses in all the men's magazines in her underwear, and says silly things during interviews. Or maybe you are Actress B, who does a range of films, from serious indies to comedies; has a no-nudity clause in all her contracts; and has a charity that she is passionate about. What are your automatic assumptions about each actress?

The same idea applies to social media. If you are always posting inconsequential statuses and goofy photos, people will think of you as silly. You might be more serious minded in real life, but today people form opinions of us based on our social media activity. Take a good look at your profile and what you post. If you were a stranger, what assumptions would you make about you? What is your online reputation?

Consider posting content that has value. By that, I mean content that interests and intrigues people and keeps them coming back for more. Regram a beautiful photo instead of posting another cat photo or a silly picture of your roommate. Link to an interesting article instead of posting what you ate for breakfast. (Unless what you ate was a work of art!) Celebrate your friends' or family members' accomplishments instead of always talking about yourself.

And remember: It's never too late to rehabilitate your online image. Start today. You don't have to delete your accounts and start over. That's kind of drastic, but you can certainly do that if you want. Maybe just clean things up a little. Delete some photos or questionable content. It might take people some time to accept the new you, but they will eventually.

ONLINE PERSONA DOS AND DON'TS

Do post things that enhance your reputation, not detract from it.

Do think before you post. Ask yourself: "How does this make me look?"

Do realize that everything you post contributes to how people view you.

Don't be one person in the real world and a different person in the digital world. People will be confused.

IS IT TIME FOR A DIGITAL DETOX?

If you haven't heard this term before, I'm happy to explain it. A digital detox means stepping away from all things social media and technology related to give your brain and psyche a break! Think about it. We're on our phones and computers constantly. Being plugged in 24/7, the way so many of us are, isn't healthy. Sometimes we need a little vacation from all things virtual. It's no different from going on a juice fast or a healthy diet if we've binged on junk food or eaten unhealthily for too long, or exercising after a period of sitting on our butts.

I go on a digital detox at least four times a month because I need to disconnect. I remove myself from the obligation to constantly update what's going on in my life as a way to refresh my brain. It's a nice mental break and I find that I feel incredibly replenished and peaceful afterward. They last one or two days at most and usually take place over a weekend.

I don't think people realize how noisy the digital world can be. It's loud out there! When you are in a calm place with no devices, it gives you the opportunity to connect with yourself as a person. You aren't letting a device dictate what you should and shouldn't be doing. There are

Let's play a game: Want a free meal :)? Make all your friends stack their phones on the table (and include yours, too). Whoever picks up the phone first pays. Happy chatting!

no notifications urging you to drop everything and see the latest text, e-mail, or comment.

Can you put away your phone for a day? Does the idea scare you? Does it make you physically sick to put your phone in a drawer for a few hours or walk away from your laptop for an afternoon? Then you are definitely a candidate for a detox!

I know many of you have jobs that revolve around the Internet these days, so the concept of a digital detox is hard to comprehend. Maybe you make a living off Etsy, maybe you're a community manager for a brand, or maybe you have customers who expect to reach you twenty-four hours a day. How can you virtually shut down when your livelihood depends on being plugged in? A digital detox isn't about going cold turkey for long periods of time (although you can do that if you want!). It's more like short periods of fasting. It's a way for you to focus on yourself and your spirit.

There are apps and services that allow you to schedule a post in advance. So if you have a sale, new video, blog post, or whatnot coming up, but you want to take a detox on that day, just schedule it in and have the app/service update for you instead!

So where do you begin? A great place to start is mealtime. Is a smartphone your most frequent dining companion? Let's change that. When you eat a meal, whether by yourself or with others, turn the ringer off and put your phone away. For the entire meal! No Foursquare check-in, no peeking at e-mail between courses or taking pictures of your tacos and posting them on Instagram. If your friends take out their phones, that's okay. It's your fast, not theirs. Maybe you like to eat in front of your computer. So many people who work in offices are guilty of that. Why don't you eat outside? Or shut down your computer and listen to some music on your headphones while you eat your sandwich, instead of surfing the Web between bites? If you eat in front of your computer at home, just shut it down. Again, put on some music, or eat in front of a window and look outside. Don't cheat and eat in front of your television as a replacement!

> ### ESTABLISH BOUNDARIES EARLY
> Make sure you keep your personal life and your work life distinct. If you're an entrepreneur and work for yourself, it's hard. I know that from personal experience. I'm completely guilty of this. It's also hard if you have a very demanding job and/or boss. But you need separation and boundaries; otherwise you won't be leading a very healthy existence. If you constantly answer your e-mail after work and on your days off, your boss and colleagues will start to view that as normal. If you don't, eventually they won't expect it from you. If you have trouble finding that separation, a few well-planned digital detoxes could be helpful.

I know this isn't easy, especially when we're so used to constant multi-tasking. If you're part of the digital generation, your smartphone is practically an extension of your hand. But it will get easier with time. Your mind will start to be clearer and you'll look forward to these breaks.

If you prefer, do it for longer periods of time, like an entire day. Maybe you can do Cyber-Free Sunday, or Monday, or any other day of the week. It's ambitious, but go for it. You might need to schedule a few periods throughout the day where you check your phone. You don't want to worry anyone if you are unreachable. Pre-detox, you can warn your friends and family, post a note on your Facebook page, or set an auto-response on your e-mail: "Hi, everybody. I'm doing a digital detox today. I won't be responding until tomorrow." Chances are, you will inspire your friends to do their own detox.

When I was in Thailand a few years ago for my first real vacation in years, I did a major digital detox. For two weeks, I only went online twice, and that was just to say hi to my family, send them some pictures, and let them know I was alive. That was it! I can barely explain how light and refreshed I felt. I had a sense of freedom I hadn't experienced in a very, very long time. The Internet is always "open" and evolving, and my job requires me to be constantly updating and creating content. I'll admit that all the digital demands can be draining. They can affect your physical and mental health and your creativity if you don't take a break.

You're not a robot. If you don't shut off, you're going to burn yourself out. I don't want that to happen to you.

ONLINE NEGATIVITY

It's easy to engage in this kind of behavior. I'm talking about anonymous comments and negative comments. There are so many opportunities to hide behind the cloak of invisibility the Internet offers, but I urge you to take the high road. Just because you can say something negative doesn't mean you should. The Internet can be an ugly place when nasty comments get thrown around, but it can also be a supportive, nurturing place.

Even though you're just one person, you'd be amazed at how much influence you can have by being a positive force online.

DIGITAL DETOX DOS AND DON'TS

Do start small. It's like running a marathon. You have to train before you run all those miles.

Do put your phone away and do shut down your computer. You can do it!

Don't set yourself up for defeat. If you have a big project coming up or lots of friends coming to town, it might be a bad time for a digital detox.

Do warn your family and closest friends. You don't want them to worry if they can't reach you.

Do enjoy the silence. Use this time to refresh and reconnect. Your brain will thank you.

Don't beat yourself up if you can't break free from your devices. Our phones and computers are big parts of our lives today. Start with small breaks of five minutes or so and build up to longer periods of time.

HOW DO I MAKE MY VIDEOS?

This is probably the number one question I get asked. The answer is that it depends on the video. I've made everything from an elaborate video in Paris with a big budget, a big crew, and lots of equipment to a simple video with just myself and my laptop. In fact, the first video I ever made was recorded on my laptop's webcam and edited with iMovie, the program that came already loaded on my MacBook Pro.

Today, I use one of three editing programs. When I'm working on a simple project or I need to edit fast, I use iMovie. If I want more control and want to jazz it up, I use Final Cut Pro X, which is like iMovie on steroids. If I want to work with other people and have them help me edit, I use Adobe Premiere, because it's easier to share and transfer video projects.

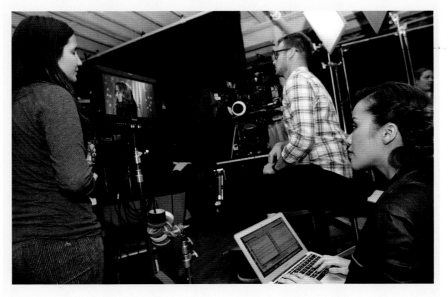

HOW TO BE TECH SMART FOR FREE

When people want to make their own videos, take better pictures, or learn different aspects of using the Internet, they ask me what classes they should take. The truth is you don't need any classes. Sure, if you have the money, go ahead. But today it's easier than ever to teach yourself how to use different programs and master various technologies. How do I know? I'm completely self-taught.

Modern computer programs are designed to be easy to use. Generally, you can just hover your arrow or cursor over a tool or icon and an explanation will pop up. Also, there are plenty of online articles and YouTube videos with hints, tips, and tricks. You just need to Google to find them. And the bonus? They're all free!

Computer programs are already expensive to purchase, so you don't want to spend *more* money just to master them. If you bought a program or have it already loaded in your laptop, just open it and give yourself a day to play. It's like learning to drive. It's one thing to learn from someone else while you sit in the passenger seat, but if you give yourself a giant open road or an empty parking lot, you'll learn faster and be more confident. I find that I'm a better learner when I just experiment.

Once you've explored on your own, head over to YouTube and browse through the tutorials. I just typed in the words "how to use iMovie," for example, and more than seven hundred thousand results came up. There are so many tutorials to choose from for every program and they exist at every level—beginner, intermediate, and advanced.

PICTURES OF YOU—AND VIDEO TOO!

As much as I love technology, there's something very nice about having printouts of your favorite photos. It's reassuring to know you have those memories on paper in case anything happens to your computer or hard drives. Actual photos also make really nice presents. A lot of people don't bother printing their photos anymore, so your friends and family will be really touched that you took the time to do this.

On the flip side, if you have old family photos, why not have them scanned? This way, you can have them forever. They won't age or warp or fade, like actual photos do. You don't have to worry about losing them to fire, theft, or time. Same thing with family movies. My mom recently found a VHS tape of my school play from kindergarten. We went from store to store looking for a VHS player. We finally found one at an electronics store, but it was $400. The video was cute, but that was a lot of money just to watch one video a few times. I found a shop that would transfer tapes to DVD format, so I had all of our family videos transferred. You definitely want to stay on top of technology. You don't want to wake up and find out you can't access precious memories because technology has moved on.

TECH-SMART DOS AND DON'TS

Don't be a digital dinosaur. Make sure you understand basic programs and tasks (creating a document, editing a picture, making a spreadsheet, etc.) or you might be left behind at work and at school.

Don't be afraid of technology. Different programs might seem complicated, but most of them are actually designed to be easy to learn and master.

Do experiment. You won't learn if you don't play around with technology. It's like makeup in the sense that you can experiment all you want. No one has to see what you create as part of the learning process except you!

Do search YouTube for free tutorials. Why pay for classes when there are so many great tutorials for free?

MY TECH MUST-HAVES

I love new equipment as much as the next person, but you don't need dozens of tech pieces to be creative. These are a couple of things I can't live without:

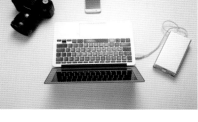

- **My laptop**
- **My phone**
- **My camera**

I can achieve anything with these three things.

DIGITAL HOUSEKEEPING

Confession time. My desktop is a big mess. I'm a total digital hoarder. I know I should be more organized and take time to straighten everything up. I'm trying to have better desktop-maintenance habits and I'm happy to report that I'm making some progress.

It's no different from taking care of your bedroom or your office. If everything is dirty and disorganized, you won't be able to find anything.

Where is that magazine you swear you saved? Who knows! It's the same as that photo you dragged from that website a few months ago. Now, where did it go? Is it with all those other photos? Or did you move it to iPhoto or throw it in a random untitled folder? Hmm . . .

Let's pledge to have better desktop habits right now. It's really like anything else. If you do something on a regular basis, it becomes a habit, like taking off your makeup each night or doing the dishes.

When I do take the time to organize my desktop, I feel so much better. People used to say, "Cluttered desk, cluttered mind," and now that applies to digital desktops. I usually force myself to clean my desktop once a month. I dedicate the time to making folders and dragging all the random photos, music, and documents into them. I always feel better when I finish, and my computer runs more smoothly. It's actually very therapeutic. I find that weekends are a great time to do this, and it's nice to start the week with a clean computer.

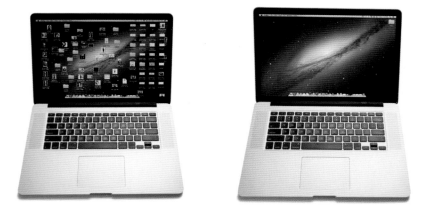

I am good about backing things up to a hard drive. Do you do that? If so, great. If not, what would you do if your computer was stolen? (That happened to me! My laptop was stolen right out of my trunk after I had my car valet parked. When I discovered the theft, my heart sank. I hadn't backed anything up and lost so many photos and videos. Lesson learned.) Or what if it mysteriously and permanently crashed? How would you get all your photos, songs, videos, and documents back? You can buy a small hard drive today for less than $100 and back everything up. It's a simple process and it shouldn't scare you. I've filled up multiple hard drives over the years with all my material and I have them stacked up with labels indicating what's on where.

DIGITAL HOUSEKEEPING DOS AND DON'TS

Do schedule time to clean up your desktop. A messy desktop slows down both your brain and your computer!

Do keep your hardware clean. When is the last time you cleaned your screen and your keyboard? Shut off your computer and wipe it down.

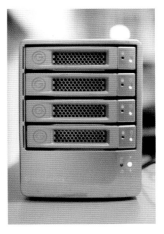

Do get in the habit of filing digital photos, documents, music, videos, and other material in the appropriate places on a regular basis.

Don't beat yourself up for digital hoarding. Your memories are important! Just be organized about them.

Do invest in an external hard drive and back things up. You'll be grateful if your computer is stolen or dies.

Do transfer old family photos and movies to more current formats. It will preserve them for future generations, and that's very special.

VIRTUAL REALITY

Technology is a magical, wonderful thing. Used correctly, it can change people's lives. It changed mine, after all. Just remember not to let technology rule your existence. Life isn't lived through a computer screen. Life is lived by having experiences, creating things, and going out and seeing the world—even just your small corner of it. Every now and then, log off and live it up.

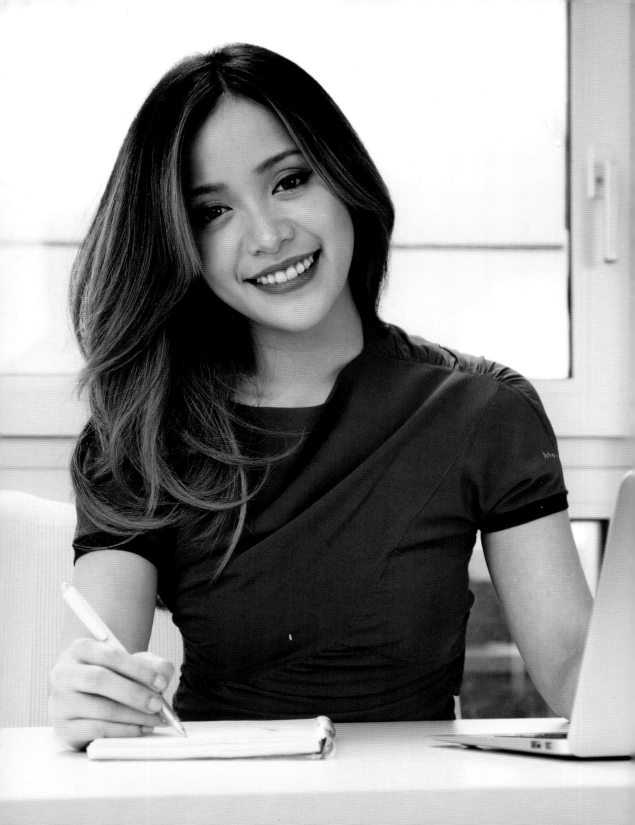

FIND (AND KEEP) A JOB YOU LOVE

don't like to make assumptions about anything—especially people. But I'm going to guess that:

you have a job

OR

you want a job

OR

one day you will need a job

If not, who are you? I'll come hang out on your desert island!

Seriously, we're going to talk about jobs—how to find a job, how to keep a job, and how to excel at your job. We'll talk résumés, communicating with current and future bosses, and more. Depending on where you are in your life and/or career, you might want to skip ahead or around in this chapter. You will spend so many hours working throughout your lifetime that you owe it to yourself to think long and hard about your career path. Many people just float into jobs, but it is possible to find a job that truly reflects you, your creativity, and what matters to you in life. People who love what they do are the luckiest people in the world.

I'm certainly not a career coach, so the information that follows is a combination of my experiences plus things I've learned from the amazing people I've worked with over the past few years. I talked to many of them about careers and what makes a good, smart employee, so I hope you enjoy reading what they shared with me. All of us can learn a lot from this chapter!

WHAT DO YOU WANT TO DO FOR A LIVING?

Does this question drive you crazy? It starts when you are a little kid with "What do you want to be when you grow up?" and then it never ends. It's cute when a five-year-old says, "I want to be an astronaut," but it's less cute—actually, really frustrating—when you are older and have no idea what you want to do. Not knowing your calling is stressful, but you're not alone. A lot of people are in the same boat.

As for me, I always wanted to be an artist. I started drawing on blank walls with crayons when I was little, and the desire to draw and create never left me. My mom, however, had other plans. She wanted me to work in the medical field. I enrolled in the health academic program at my technical high school and became an expert on bones, CPR, etc. (Bet you didn't know that about me!) These were useful things to learn, so I'm happy to have that knowledge. But I knew deep down this wasn't my passion.

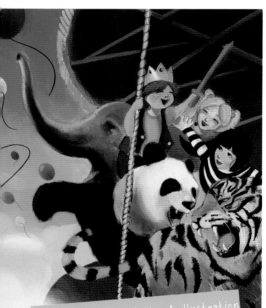
I drew this for my children's illustration class. I wanted to capture the laughter and imagination of kids.

In my senior year, we had to pick the profession we wanted to pursue and shadow someone with that job. For whatever reason, I selected X-ray technician, so I followed a radiology technician around the local hospital for two weeks. He had a portable X-ray machine and we would run to different parts of the hospital to X-ray patients, just like in a TV show—except this was real life. There were so many people in pain and he told me all these crazy stories that I don't even want to repeat. I felt traumatized—and I wasn't the one with the actual trauma!

I realized I couldn't spend the rest of my life doing this. I did not have the guts to be in that industry and to handle the mental stress. I'm too emotional. No one needs a radiology tech, or a doctor or nurse, who is always bursting into tears.

I could have forced myself to do what my mother wanted and made a nice, stable living, but I would have been miserable. I've seen how unhappy some of my family members have been with their careers, my mom included, and how they suffered because of it. I said to myself, "I never want to be that person. I'd rather be happy, even if I don't make a lot of money." So right then and there, at the age of seventeen, I realized that I needed to change direction. I was going to become an artist. I would disappoint my mother, which pained me greatly, but I knew that in time she would understand.

There's a lot of honor in doing a job, working hard, and giving it your all. But you owe it to yourself to uncover your hidden talents or a passion that can be turned into a profession. If you already know what that is, congratulations! You can jump ahead. If not, read on. . . .

So what are you good at? "Nothing" is not an option! Everyone is good at something, but they don't always realize it. You just need to find that thing. Ask your friends, ask a family member, or ask a teacher, professor, or mentor what he or she thinks you are good at. Someone else might see something in you that you don't.

If you truly think you're not good at anything, let me ask you some questions:

- What do you love?
- Do you have a hobby or an activity that you do all the time?
- Is there anything that excites you? A TV show, a sport, a book, a computer game, a fashion brand?

Any of these things can be turned into a profession. How? The answer may not be obvious and might require a lot of Google searches, but that's okay. We'll figure it out. When I decided to follow my heart and become an artist, I knew I was about to put myself on a difficult path. Have you ever heard the term *starving artist*? That exists for a reason. It's really hard to make a living as an artist! I calculated how much money I would need to pay my rent, buy groceries and art supplies, make car payments, and have a little bit left over for fun. I started researching which jobs in the art field paid in that range. (There are plenty of websites that feature salary information, such as CareerPath.com and LinkedIn.) I came up with illustration, computer animation, and graphic design. I decided I would pursue a career in one of those areas.

Let's say you love TV or film. I'm not exaggerating when I say there are thousands of career options related to these fields, from operating cameras to writing scripts, representing actors and actresses, assisting directors, designing sets, and working at a cable company. Take a good look at the credits next time you are watching a TV show or movie. Each line represents a different job.

Same thing with sports. There are athletes, coaches, sports doctors, physical therapists, sports journalists and bloggers, venue managers, licensed merchandise producers, and on and on. Same with tech. Same with fashion.

Once you scratch the surface, a lot of things will reveal themselves. If you zero in on a particular job, find someone who has that job and figure out how he or she got there. Maybe there's an article about him or her online. Maybe he or she is on Twitter or Facebook and you can send a tweet or post something asking how he or she got his or her start. You're not asking this person for anything except a little advice. It might surprise you, but I've found that many people will take the time to tell you about their career. Reaching out to a stranger might require getting out of your comfort zone and not being shy, especially if that's how you are naturally. But go for it! Usually, when you put something out into the universe, you get something back.

THE INFORMATIONAL INTERVIEW

Have you ever heard of this? An informational interview can be very useful as you decide what to do with your life or as you continue along your career path. It's not a job interview. It's a meeting that you request with someone in order to learn more about his or her job or career and how he or she got where he or she is. You can ask someone you know for an informational interview, or you can take a chance and ask someone you don't know but admire. They won't always say yes. (Don't hold it against them, especially if you're a stranger to them!) But I know many successful executives who take the time to do informational interviews because it's part of giving back, so there's a chance they could say yes.

You can do informational interviews at any point in your life and career—before you have a job, while you're in college, when you're considering a career change.

How do you get an informational interview? Send a nice letter or e-mail. If the recipient says yes, do your homework before the interview. Research him or her online and come prepared with smart questions. Keep the interview limited to thirty to forty-five minutes. Explain where you are in your career and why you wanted the chance to learn more about him or her. You can take notes if you like. Remember, this is not the time to ask for a job. But you can ask how he or she got *his or her* job. Don't leave without asking if he or she has any advice for you.

Make sure to send the interviewer a handwritten thank-you note!

HOW TO FIND YOUR FIRST JOB

Okay: You need a job, but you've never had one. How do you even begin? It can be very daunting when you are starting from scratch.

I remember when I applied for the job at the Lancôme counter. (Remember that from the first chapter? Maybe it's not a great story to remind you about because I didn't get the job!) It was scary walking into the department store and being interviewed by someone I had never met before.

I had no résumé and I didn't have the experience they were looking for. And then no one called to tell me I didn't get the job. It was a bummer all around. I wouldn't find another job until I got work as a waitress.

What could I have done differently? Nothing, really. I just wasn't the right person for the job. My only previous experience was working as a hostess at a restaurant, so maybe I should have focused on restaurants or food-service jobs. It's not bad to reach for the stars sometimes; you just might grab one. And if not, at least you tried. The more job interviews you go on, the better you get at the process. You'll be less nervous and you'll know what to expect.

Here are some tips for how to find that first job:

- Hit the Web: Go to your favorite search engine and type in the word *job* and the name of your hometown or nearest city. Start clicking and see what's out there.

- Get social: Put a twist on the "help wanted" ad with your own "job wanted" ad. Go on Twitter or your Facebook page and let the world know you are looking for a job. Be serious rather than jokey. You never know who will respond with some advice, suggestions, or an actual job. If you have a good relationship with your principal or dean, or any professors or teachers, tell them you are looking. Tell your friends, your friends' parents, and your neighbors. You never know. You can accomplish a lot via word of mouth.

- Be old-school: Look for a job the old-fashioned way. Go where the stores are in your community and see if they have Help Wanted signs in the windows. Walk in and ask about the job or ask to see the manager. Make sure to look presentable and be polite. Some places, like the mall, won't have signs in the window. Just walk in and ask for the manager and ask if there are any job openings. If it's a chain store, the manager might have you fill out an application even if a job isn't available at that moment. Fill it out anyway (and write neatly). You have nothing to lose. Maybe someone will quit or get promoted tomorrow and they will have an opening! Make sure to have pertinent information with you, like your Social Security number and the name and number of a reference, in case you're asked for it.

- See what your options are: When you're first starting out and you have no experience, you can't be picky. You might have to take your expectations down a notch. See what jobs are available and see what the requirements are. Look for "help wanted" ads that say "no experience required" or "willing to train." If it says "experience required," you might want to keep looking.

- Go ahead and apply: If you are applying in person, you should always be polite. This extends to how you look. Be mindful of the environment and dress appropriately. Working for an accountant is different from working for a rock star, so consider that when you are deciding between a nice top with a skirt and some leather leggings with a ripped-up shirt.

> ### WHAT'S A REFERENCE?
> A reference is a person who can tell your potential employer something about you. Maybe it's your last boss, a teacher or professor, or a friend who already works at the company where you are looking for a job. You will need a reference for most jobs, so make sure you have somebody who will say nice things about you! You should never give someone's name and contact information as a reference without asking him or her first. Just ask nicely: "Do you mind if I use you as a reference?" Make sure you don't ask the boss who fired you or the teacher who doesn't like you.

If you need to fill out an application, write everything neatly and accurately and double-check what you've written. Imagine if you wrote the wrong phone number or e-mail address, or it was so illegible they read it incorrectly. You might wonder why they never called. And make sure to proofread it before turning it in. Proofreading means checking anything you've written for grammar, punctuation, and spelling mistakes. If proofreading isn't your strength, try reading what you've written out loud. Sometimes that is helpful. (If you need to proofread a document you've created through Google or Word, or another program, use whatever spelling-and-grammar-check tool is available.) You could also have a friend or colleague check it. A second pair of eyes might catch things you don't notice.

If there is no form to fill out and you need to send an e-mail inquiring about the job, keep it brief and to the point. Say a little about who you are, why you want the job, and how you can be reached. You want it to read more like a letter than a text message.

If you know the name of the person to whom you are writing, use his or her name. If not, use "To Whom It May Concern." Each situation will be different, obviously, but here are two examples:

To Whom It May Concern:

I am writing to apply for the job of dishwasher at the Corner Café. I am a senior at Thomas Jefferson High School and belong to the art club. My family moved here from Seattle last year. I am a hard worker and would like to be part of the team at your restaurant. I can be reached at 555-321-1234 or at this e-mail address. Thank you.

Sincerely,
Tom Smith

Dear Ms. Jones,

I would like to apply for the job of receptionist at the New Wave Salon. I am a part-time student at the state university. I love the fast-paced atmosphere at hair salons and I am an excellent multitasker. I can be reached at 555-321-1234 or at this e-mail address. Thank you.

Sincerely,
Jane Wu

Before you hit send, read the e-mail several times and don't forget to use your grammar-and-spell-check option. If finding mistakes isn't your strong suit, have a friend read the e-mail for you.

- Use your common sense: Be careful when applying for jobs that sound too good to be true. They probably are! There are plenty of scams out there—things like telemarketing jobs that promise tons of money, except you work on commission (that's where you only get paid when you actually sell something). You also might run into things that would make you compromise your beliefs. Maybe you'd need to use heavy-handed selling tactics, or sell things to people who don't need them, or even do something illegal or unethical. I always say:

Trust your instincts

Trust your gut

Trust *yourself*

If something doesn't feel right, it's not right for *you*. Move on. Something else will come along.

NEED EXPERIENCE?
MAYBE YOU HAVE IT ALREADY

When you have no experience, it can be really hard to find a job. That's why I didn't get the job at the Lancôme counter. The woman who interviewed me even said, "It's too bad you don't have any experience." I told her I knew I could do the job, but that wasn't enough.

You can't get a job without experience, but how can you get experience without a job?

Well, let's take a look at how you spend the day. Do you do any of the following?

Babysit
Laundry
Lawn work
Drive your grandmother to her appointments
Play sports
Coach or manage any teams
Belong to any clubs or organizations
Social media
Write
Photography
Build websites
Make videos

Don't shortchange yourself. You might have job experience and not even realize it. A lot of these things, especially clubs and school activities, can count as job experience.

If you answered no to all of the things above, you might want to join some clubs or organizations at school or in your community—quick! These are great ways to get experience without having an actual job. Managing your college basketball team, working for a school or local paper, doing audiovisual work for a local play, writing the weekly bulletin for your church—all of these count as experience. You might not get paid, but you learn and develop skills that you can mention to a potential employer, like accountability, time management, working with other people, and problem solving. Activities like this also help prove that you are a responsible person.

HOW ABOUT VOLUNTEERING?

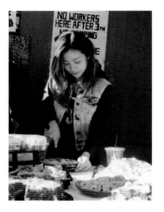

Volunteering is a great way to gain experience when you can't find a job. Remember, volunteers work for free and do it because they care about the organization or cause at hand. You do not want to be a halfhearted volunteer. That is not fair to the organization. But if you have time and really want to help, volunteering is something you'll never regret. You might even make a difference in someone's life, and nothing is greater than that.

Where to start? Think of a cause that's important to you and see what the volunteer opportunities are in your community. You'll be surprised at the range of options. You can give your time at an animal rescue center, a soup kitchen, an after-school tutoring program, and on and on.

LET'S TALK ABOUT INTERNSHIPS

Where do we even begin? Internships are such a big deal these days. You know what they are, right? An internship is where you work for a person or a company to gain experience. It's almost like what an apprenticeship was centuries ago. You might not get paid, you might get minimum wage, or you might do it in exchange for college credit. The goal is for you to gain on-the-job training, find out more about a particular profession, learn from the employees, and walk away with either a job offer or some good references.

Internships can be hard to get because everyone wants a good internship to put on his or her résumé. If you don't want an internship and you are still in school, you *should* want one! It could make all the difference when you are finished with your studies and looking for a "real" job. These days, when competing for top jobs in many fields, it's not enough to have a good education. You need to have a good internship, or even two or three.

You should come up with an internship plan for yourself. Most internships are meant for college students and recent college graduates, so you should plan to have internships during that period in your life. And please note that the most competitive internships require that you apply months in advance, so don't wait until the last minute. It is feasible that you could get an internship if you are in high school or if you've been out of college and are looking to switch careers, but it will be harder than when you are an actual college student.

So where do you start? Should you send your résumé to *InStyle*, Instagram, or H&M? Maybe, maybe not. Internships are very competitive at the most famous places. You should look at applying for internships the way you looked at applying to college:

- What do you want to specialize in? Pick the field in which you want to work. If you're a premed major, it might be hard to find an internship in television, unless of course you explain that you want to be a doctor on a news TV show or talk show. A zoology major might have a hard time getting an internship at a fashion company. Be realistic. Or have a talk with yourself and make sure you're majoring in a field that really interests you.

- What can you afford? Do you live in a small town without many resources? Do you work to put yourself through school? Can you move to a big city for a summer? Your answers to these questions are going to dictate the when, where, and what of your internship. If money is an issue, you're going to need an internship that is either local, part-time, or paid. If you want an internship that is based out of town, don't forget you'll need a place to live. Some colleges offer summer housing for interns regardless of whether they go to that school. It's more affordable than an apartment, especially in expensive cities like New York, San Francisco, and London. Look into it.

- How do you find out about available internships? Start online. There are so many websites about internships. You'll find a wealth of information on them from a variety of companies, plus helpful tips on how to apply.

If you are in college, visit the career services office or center. They might post information about available internships. Chances are, the college has relationships with certain companies, organizations, and alumni who help facilitate internships. It's not uncommon for a company to regularly hire interns from one college—as long as the last intern from that school was a good one!

Ask people. Just start telling friends, fellow students, relatives, etc., that you're looking for an internship. Everybody knows somebody. You might just find a lead this way.

Last, put the word out on social media. Let it be known that you are looking for an internship. Mention the field you are interested in, city or town, and time period.

- Cold call! Do you know what that term means? It means getting in touch with someone whom you don't know and who doesn't know you. Looking for a magazine internship? Pick up your favorite magazine and look for the names of the editors. (There's usually a list in the front of the magazine with the names of everyone who works there. It's called a masthead.) Love a certain TV show? Get the names of the crew from the credits. You might find these people via Twitter or LinkedIn.

What do you do next? If they're on Twitter, send a simple tweet saying, "Do you mind directing me to the person in charge of internships at your company? Thank you!" Or if you have their e-mail address, send an e-mail that says:

Dear [fill in the name],

I'm very interested in working at [fill in the name of the company]. Do you mind telling me who is in charge of the internship program so I can get in touch with him or her? Thank you in advance for your assistance.

Best,
[Fill in your name]

Don't be a stalker, though! There's a fine line between a nice, polite tweet or LinkedIn e-mail and going overboard. Don't send any e-mail correspondence more than twice and keep social media interaction limited to one post or tweet. No response? Move on.

- What is human resources? This is a term you need to know. All big companies have a human resources (or HR) department that is in charge of hiring (and, gulp, firing) people. Chances are, if a company has an HR department, it oversees the internship program. You might have your first interview with someone from HR. If you get the internship, you might have to check in with the HR representative from time to time during your internship.

  If you have your heart set on an internship with a certain company, find its website and look for a jobs tab or section. There might be an e-mail address for the HR department or employment inquiries. Or, think old-school! Pick up the phone, call the company, and ask who is in charge of internships, or ask for the HR department. Use some detective work! It will pay off.

- What is your dream internship? Think of this like your "reach" college. You know what that is, right? It's a school that is slightly out of your league because of the required GPA, or money, or some other factor, but you really, really would like to go there one day. So you apply. It's okay to dream big for internships too. You never know. The company might see something in you that they really like.

- Can you apply off-season? Everyone wants a summer internship, but many companies offer internships year-round. Can you intern during the school year instead of the summer? The competition isn't as intense and you might have an easier time snagging a top internship. But there's a catch. It means balancing all your required classes, your social life, and perhaps a paid job with your internship. Or it means you need to take a semester's leave from school. Consider whether this option works for you.

- No internships in your town? This is a reality for a lot of people. My Florida college town was not filled with awesome internship options, so I know what it's like. You need to think out of the box. Maybe there are businesses in town that would love an intern but never had the time or energy to put a program in place or even look for an intern. Get in touch with them and explain what you would like to do. Is there a small radio or TV station in town? A company that builds websites? A restaurant that needs help with social media? It might take a little work, but you can create your own opportunity.

YOUR INTERNSHIP GOALS

If you are fortunate enough to get an internship, you need to take it seriously. You are there to learn, not just to kill time and get something on your résumé. I want you to focus on the following things during your internship, which in turn will improve your chances of securing a full-time job when the time comes:

- Learn everything you can: Be a sponge. Interns occupy a special place that entry-level employees don't, so use the opportunity to ask questions, shadow people, and master a range of tasks. When you're a full-time employee, people expect you to know about your job and to do the exact job you were hired for. But when you're an intern, everyone knows you are there to learn. The company's employees might be more interested in sharing information with you about the workplace, their careers, and how to succeed etc.

    Just don't be too eager or annoying. Again, fine line! Have good situational awareness. If everyone in the room is quiet and typing away, maybe it's not a good time to ask all your questions. It's important to scope out the scene. Lunch breaks are a great opportunity to drop by and ask a question. Usually, that's the time when people are checking their personal e-mails, making calls, etc. Ask your questions, be mindful of their time, and absorb as much as you can!

- Work hard: This seems obvious, but a lot of interns are slackers. Be the intern who knows how to do things and whom everyone comes to rely upon. You want to be seen as someone of value, meaning that you are a team player. Do your job with excellence. It will be appreciated, believe me.

- Accept small tasks graciously: You will be asked to do things that aren't very glamorous—filing papers, stuffing envelopes, fetching coffee, answering phones. Don't underestimate the task at hand. You are being tested. Your boss wants to see if you can handle basic tasks. If you can't do the little things perfectly, you will not be given bigger things to do. Most people start at the bottom. Remember that, and don't give attitude. Many people would be grateful to have the opportunity to do the work you are doing. Tuck that in the back of your mind whenever you're feeling down. It will all pay off in the long run.

- Make sure everyone knows your name: This might seem obvious too, but at big companies, there are so many people and so many interns coming through season after season that people might not remember your name. Don't be afraid to remind people what your name is. Say, "Hi, I'm [your name]," when you pop your head in their offices. Eventually, they'll say, "I know who you are!" Heck, wear a nameplate necklace. You want to stand out—for the right reasons.

  Don't slink in and slink out of the workplace. At the start of each day, walk past your boss's office and say good morning. A friendly gesture goes a long way! Before you leave at night, ask if there's anything else he or she needs, and if not, say good night. This is all part of making a good impression.

  When you finish your internship, you want to be able to use your boss as a reference. Six months later, or even a year or two later, when someone calls your former boss and says, "[Your name] would like to work for our company and

Here I am working with design students on em cosmetics packaging. I have always believed that art students are fearless and bold with their creativity.

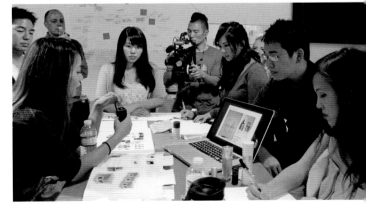

I'm calling to see if she was a good employee," you want him or her to say, "Oh, [your name] was awesome," not "Who?"

WHEN YOUR INTERNSHIP IS OVER

Leave on the date you agreed upon when you started, never before! Are you leaving on good terms with your boss? Will you be able to use him or her as a reference? Yes and yes? Great!

Next, you need to ask yourself, "Is this a place I would like to work?" If the answer is yes, ask if you can have an exit interview with your immediate boss or your point person from human resources. Maybe they already know you would like to work there, but this is your last chance to make it official. Sit down with them, tell them you would like to work there one day, and ask if they think you would be a good candidate.

If you are looking for immediate employment, ask if there are any job openings. Don't be shy! You worked hard and you want to know what your options are. There's nothing wrong with that. It never hurts to ask. You don't want to miss an opportunity because you didn't ask the right question.

Keep in touch with the people for whom and with whom you worked. Internships are where many professional relationships begin. This can help you in the future when a job opens up at the company, or if your contacts move on to bigger things. You'll automatically have a new job lead!

AN INTERNSHIP WARNING

There has been a lot of controversy lately about unpaid internships. Interns who did not get paid have turned around and sued the companies they worked for because they felt, after the fact, that they should have been compensated.

Interns should never get taken advantage of. You are there to learn, not to be someone's slave. If you feel you are being taken advantage of, whether you have a paid or unpaid internship, you should definitely speak up. Talk to your boss or the person in charge of internships. If the situation is very bad, talk to your boss's boss. The same thing goes for workplace bullying. But don't waste your boss's time if people are simply being mean. At some point during your career, you will encounter people who aren't nice to you. It's never pleasant when it happens, but you can take the high road in how you deal with these things. Often the best advice is to ignore and don't engage.

But don't confuse menial tasks with being taken advantage of. And don't complain just because you have a tough boss. As I mentioned, a lot of intern work is doing boring, basic tasks. If you can nail those, there's a good chance you'll be rewarded with more interesting work. If you can't nail them, you'll be stuck doing them until you do get them perfect. A friend of mine worked with an intern who complained on the very first day! She said she thought she would be doing more important tasks, like planning parties. Trust me, you won't be planning parties on the first day of any internship!

Last, if you're being treated in an abusive, offensive, or inappropriate manner, definitely speak up. That should not be a part of anyone's internship.

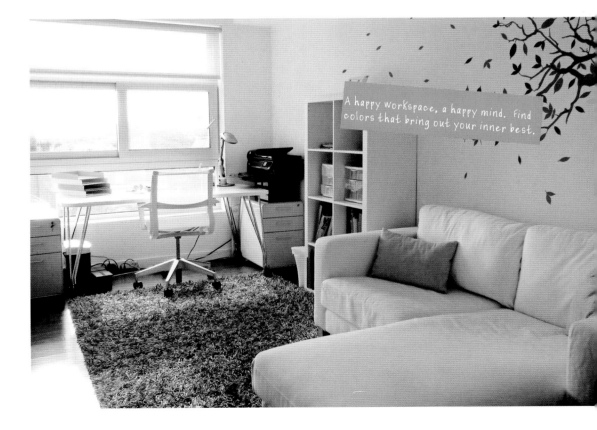

Work Rules for Everyone

Internship? First job? Fifth job? These tips will help you
be super professional at any workplace.

1. Be punctual.

2. Look the part. Many workplaces have a "look" or "uniform." Learn what that is.

3. Dress appropriately. When you bend down or kneel, are you revealing any body parts or undergarments you shouldn't be? You could be asked to file things and move items to high or low shelves, so be prepared with the right clothing.

4. Put your gadgets on vibrate or silent when at work.

5. Keep personal phone conversations and texting to an absolute minimum.

6. Don't abuse the sick-day policy.

7. Practice good grooming habits. Gross nails, greasy hair, and B.O.? Do we even need to talk about that?

8. Don't wear too much fragrance or aftershave. (Especially on a job interview!) The only person who should be able to smell you is you.

9. Don't take too many breaks. Starbucks isn't paying your salary.

10. Don't run out the door the second the workday is done.

11. Never follow your boss or add him or her on social media unless he or she follows you.

12. Do not complain about your job or your coworkers on social media. You never know who can see what you write, even if you think it's private.

13. Be wise about any Web surfing or e-mails that you send from company computers. Chances are, your employer can read and monitor everything you do.

14. Always keep your résumé updated. You never know when you will need it.

15. But . . . you should stay in most jobs a minimum of one year. If you bounce around every few months, potential employers won't hire you for fear you can't commit.

16. Always give two weeks' notice when you resign.

17. Always leave gracefully. (Good advice for everything in life!)

18. Always send a handwritten thank-you note or an e-mail after you leave a job. (But only if you resigned. Not if you were fired!)

HOW TO WRITE A COVER LETTER AND RÉSUMÉ

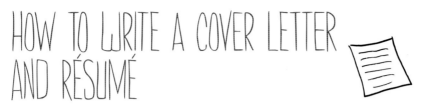

Often, a potential employer will request a résumé and cover letter. A résumé is a document that has all your information on it. Name, address, education, and work experience. A cover letter is a letter that explains who you are, what job you want, and why you are qualified for it.

For many people, writing a great résumé and cover letter is the hardest part of job hunting, but it doesn't need to be. I'm going to give you an example of each that you can use as a guide. You also can look online for different examples of good résumés and cover letters.

First, here are a few basic tips:

- Use a nice basic font. I prefer Arial, Times New Roman, Cambria—anything clean and readable.

- Make sure the size isn't too small—eleven or twelve is great. Any bigger and it looks like you're desperate to fill space. Any smaller and the recipient might struggle to read it.

- Make sure everything is spaced properly.

- Don't overdesign your résumé. (Unless you're applying for a graphic design job!)

- Use your grammar-and-spell-check function.

- Proofread for any typos or factual mistakes.

- Save each document as a PDF.

- Give each PDF a straightforward name—"Jane Smith Résumé" or "Jane Smith Cover Letter," for example.

SAMPLE COVER LETTER

Give your address.

123 Main Street
New City, NY 11111
March 15, 2015

Don't forget the date.

Who are you writing to? Name, title, employer, address.

Mary Jones
Digital Editor
New City Newspaper
456 Broadway
New City, NY 11112

Use a colon after the salutation.

Use Mr. or Ms.

Dear Ms. Jones:

Don't know whom to write to? Try "To Whom It May Concern:"

Why are you writing?

Mention the job you are applying for.

I am writing to apply for the social media intern position at the New City News-paper available this summer. Social media is a passion of mine. I am proficient in all social media platforms. I use them personally, and I am responsible for the social media activity for the track team at New City High School, where I am a senior. *Who are you?*

Tell them about some experience you have.

I post all information about upcoming track meets, as well as the track meet scores. I started a YouTube channel for the track team and post videos of the track meets, as well as interviews with each team member. I also started an Instagram account for the team and post photos of the meets and team members. *Keep it brief.*

Please hire me.

I would love the opportunity to work with you and your team and learn how a newspaper approaches social media and various digital matters. I can be reached at janesmith11@niceemail.com and am available for an interview any day after school. Thank you for your time.

Always say thank you!

When can you come in for an interview?

Sincerely,

[Signature] *Don't forget to sign your name.*

Jane Smith

Make your name a little bigger than
everything else on the page.

Jane Smith

123 Main Street
New City, NY 11111

Permanent address

(555) 555-5555 janesmith11@niceemail.com

Contact info—remember, no silly e-mail address.

Where
did/do you
work?

WORK EXPERIENCE

Main Street Coffee Shop, New City, NY
Counter clerk, January 2013 to present

When did you have the job?

- Responsible for opening the coffee shop every Saturday and Sunday for the seven a.m. start time.
- Set up the coffee and milk station each morning and keep it neatly maintained and stocked during my shift.
- Ring up customers' purchases and run credit cards or make change.
- Count out the tips for the team after our shift.
- Share responsibility for cleaning the restroom and taking out the trash.

List your
responsibilities.

Job title?

Jones Family
Babysitter, Summer 2012

Use the right tense: Job over? Past
tense. Current job? Present tense.

- Watched all three Jones children, Monday through Friday, from eight a.m. to five p.m.
- Made their breakfast, lunch, and snacks and started dinner for Mr. and Mrs. Jones.
- Escorted the children to weekly tennis lessons.

Schooling?.

EDUCATION

New City High School, New City, NY
Senior
Honor Roll student

List any honors or awards.

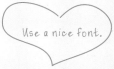

Use a nice font.

CLUBS AND ACTIVITIES

New City High School Track Team
Assistant manager, January to May 2013

Don't forget any school activities.

- Helped the manager schedule practices, travel, and track meets.
- Was responsible for transporting, packing, and unpacking all equipment needed by the team.
- Posted track meet information on social media.
- Started Instagram and YouTube accounts for the team.
- Created YouTube videos featuring the track meets and interviews with the players.

Space everything nicely so things look
balanced and not on top of each other.

SKILLS

Excellent organizational skills.
Proficient in PowerPoint, Excel, and Final Cut Pro.
Proficient in all social media platforms, including Facebook, Twitter, Instagram, Vine, and YouTube.

Got skills?
List 'em.

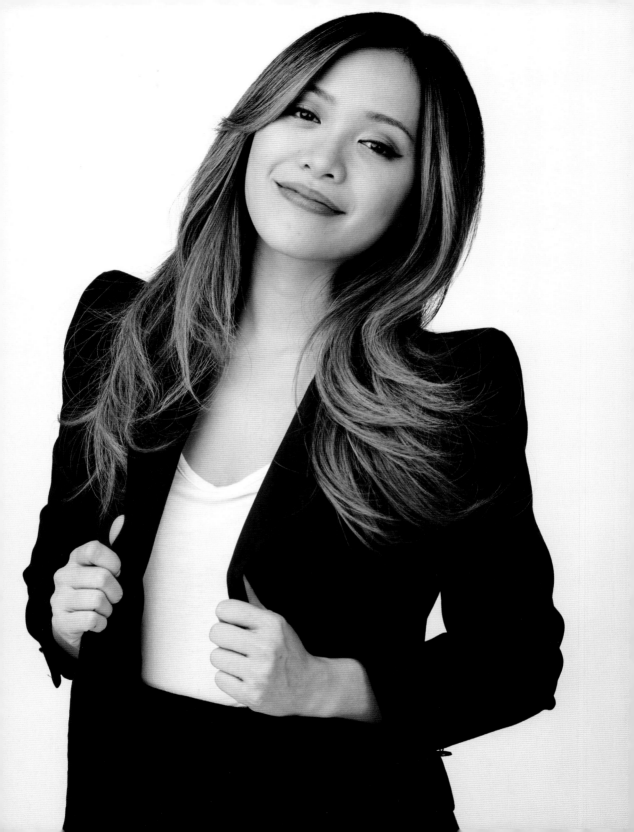

MY FAVORITE JOB-HUNTING TIP

About to apply for a job? Try mailing your letter and résumé instead of sending it via e-mail. Most people get dozens if not hundreds of work e-mails a day, but they rarely get letters. So go ahead. As long as you send a nice, professional letter and résumé, you have nothing to lose. You'll certainly stand out from the pack!

E-MAIL SMARTS

Do you have a serious e-mail address? If you're job hunting, you'd better have one. Don't even think of applying for a job if your e-mail address contains the word *sexy* or *hot*, or any suggestive numbers! Get a nice basic Gmail address with your name, or a simple variation on your name.

HOW TO NAIL AN INTERVIEW

Chances are, before you get any job or internship, you will have to go through the interview process. Depending on the job, you can have anywhere from one to ten interviews! Even a single interview can be daunting, but here are some tips for being a great interviewee.

- Be punctual and prepared: Obviously you are going to be nicely groomed and arrive early. Know the name of the person you will be meeting with and the exact address with cross streets.

- Bring a printed copy of your résumé: The interviewer probably has your résumé, so this is just a backup.

- Shake hands: When you meet the person who will be interviewing you, shake his or her hand. You don't want the handshake to be too soft or too firm. Nothing is worse than a weird, wimpy handshake—or a bone-crushing one. Practice on a friend if you have to.

- Don't be too nervous: Interviews can be nerve-wracking! I totally understand if you are nervous, but try your best to hide it and present the confident (but not overly confident) you. Fake it if you have to! Give yourself a little pep talk and do some deep breathing beforehand.

- Look them in the eye: Whoever you meet that day, look him or her in the eye when you are talking. It's okay to look away every now and then, but don't constantly avert your eyes or look at the floor. People like direct eye contact. It shows respect. But don't overdo it! You have to break eye contact every once in a while or it might get too awkward. It's an interview, not a staring contest.

- Do your homework: What do you know about the company? What do you know about the person doing the interview? Go online and do some research. Chances are, the interviewer will ask if you have any questions for him or her. Don't shake your head no. Ask some questions about the company and ask the person about him- or herself. You're not there to conduct an interrogation, but a few smart questions will help make you look good.

- Send a thank-you: Always follow up with a handwritten thank-you note mailed as soon after the interview as possible. If that's not possible (say you did the interview via Skype and you live on the other side of the world, or maybe you have the *worst* handwriting), it's okay to send an e-mail.

YOU DIDN'T GET THE JOB?

You know what the worst thing is? When you don't get the job and no one even calls to tell you! They just leave you waiting and wondering. Well, if no one calls or e-mails after a few weeks, you can assume you didn't get the job. Usually, most job interviews end with the words *We'll call if we're interested* or something to that effect.

When I didn't get the Lancôme job, my mom said to me, "Michelle, when one door closes, another will open. Just because this opportunity didn't happen doesn't mean there's not going to be another one down the line." The rejection encouraged me to make my first beauty tutorial a few days later. So you never know.

Don't get too down and don't take it personally. Just move on. Keep applying. Sometimes looking for a job can *be* a full-time job, and that's just the way it is.

I CAN'T FIND A JOB—ANYWHERE

That really stinks, and I'm so sorry. Unemployment is a reality for many people and it can be very demoralizing when you keep looking and looking and can't find anything.

There are a few things you can try. Definitely get out there and volunteer if that's a possibility. It will prevent you from having any big time gaps on your résumé. It also will show that you have initiative and that you care about your community and about others. It will give you the ability to showcase some work skills that would otherwise go unseen.

If you are between the ages of sixteen and twenty-four, check out Job Corps. This is a program administered by the U.S. Department of Labor that provides job training and placement. Go to JobCorps.gov for more information.

Maybe it's time for you to take matters into your own hands. In the next chapter, we're going to talk about how to create your own job. I'll explain how to think like an entrepreneur and *be* an entrepreneur. It's a new day, and you have more power to do your own thing than ever before!

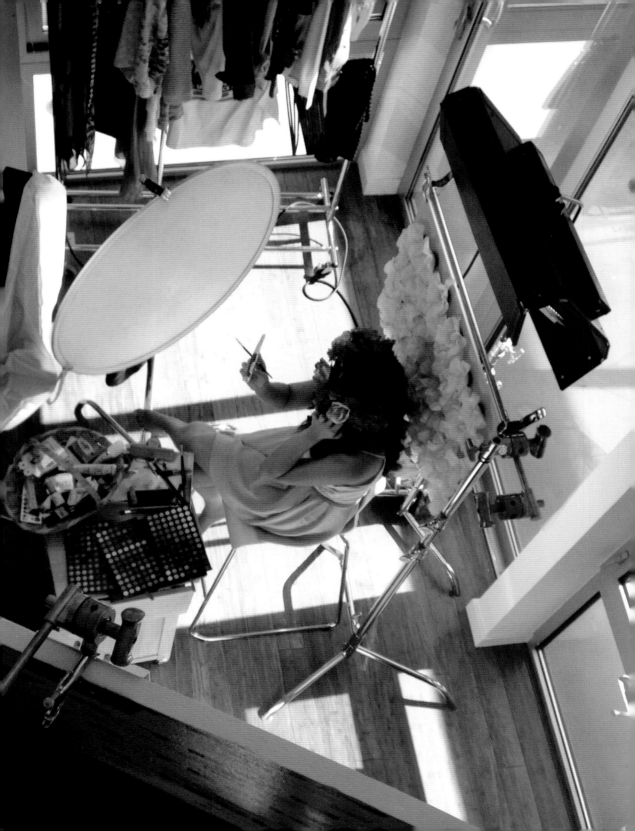

TURN YOUR PASSION INTO A PROFESSION

oesn't it seem like everyone is interested in starting his or her own business today? I think it has a lot to do with the way technology has expanded our lives and put so much power into the hands of the individual. There's also the allure of Silicon Valley and the start-up culture that resulted in Apple, Google, Facebook, and the like. The idea that you can start a business in your dorm room or your parents' garage and become a millionaire in just a few short years is very powerful. That said, the attraction isn't purely about the potential payout. I believe it's about wanting to take control of your destiny, be your own boss, and really harness your creativity.

Is this something you're considering? Do you have an idea for a business? Yes and yes? Wonderful! What if you don't? That's okay too. You never know when you'll wake up in the middle of the night with a great idea. It's good for you to understand the ins and outs of entrepreneurship. And perhaps you do have a great idea and you just don't know it. Look at me! I didn't intend to turn my hobby into my business. But I'm proof that you can turn your passion into your profession.

Whether you decide to have a small side business or take the plunge with something bigger, you won't regret it. Being an entrepreneur is a brave, amazing thing. It's one of the hardest career paths you could choose, but one of the most rewarding too. There are more tools for entrepreneurs than ever before. So many free programs are available online, and crowd-funding has removed the biggest obstacle of all: financing your biz!

I know a lot of people consider me a beauty expert, but first and foremost, I consider myself a businessperson. Here's some more about my story and the lessons I've learned.

AN ACCIDENTAL ENTREPRENEUR

I am a proud entrepreneur, yet I never set out to be my own boss. When I started making videos, I did it for fun and to teach others. In the early days, it never crossed my mind that being a vlogger on YouTube could translate into a full-time job. I went to art school thinking I would stay there for four years, graduate, and find work as a graphic designer or illustrator—for someone else! Did I ever think I would be a CEO one day? Absolutely not. Then social media exploded and changed everything.

Companies started reaching out to me, which is when I realized that vlogging could be a job. I needed to become a businessperson very quickly, and I did. I don't have an MBA from a prestigious business school, but I've learned more along the way than I ever could have in a classroom.

Today, I know dozens of other entrepreneurs and I have so much respect for them. They are artists, *macaron* makers, restaurateurs, vloggers, makeup artists, hairdressers, singers, and fashion designers. They wake up every day and work their butts off. They juggle a million tasks and do what it takes, from fixing their own plumbing to doing their own PR. They love what they do and couldn't imagine doing anything else. In many cases, they're creating jobs for other people, which is a great thing. In this chapter, we're going to talk about what it takes to be an entrepreneur, and I'll share some tips and tricks that have served me very well. Start it up!

THE ENTREPRENEURIAL PERSONALITY

It takes a very specific person to be an entrepreneur. Here are a few questions to ask yourself:

- Do you have a great idea for a business?
- Do you have lots of great ideas?
- Are you a problem solver?
- Can you handle financial instability?
- Are you a people person?
- Do you like to work hard?
- Do you have a thick skin?

You don't have to answer yes to every single one of these questions, but you should answer yes to most of them. If you didn't, this might not be the career path for you just yet. But I would never want to deter anyone or squash someone's dream, so please keep reading for tips on how to *develop* an entrepreneurial personality!

MONEY AND SACRIFICE

Unfortunately, much of being an entrepreneur often comes down to money. It's almost impossible to get a business off the ground without funding. If you want to make T-shirts or cookies or videos, at the very least you need money for supplies. Then there is all the other stuff you need money for. There are definitely ways to be scrappy and resourceful. You can build your own website. You can forgo business cards. But what about living expenses, such as car payments, rent, and groceries? Well, there's always the bus, your parents' house, and instant ramen!

Most of the entrepreneurs I know held down one or even two jobs that helped them pay the bills while they laid the groundwork for their businesses. They didn't shop for fun stuff, they didn't eat out, they didn't get a lot of sleep, and they lived with multiple roommates. They put every dime they made toward their fledgling companies. Are you ready for that?

There are lots of ways to finance your dreams. Maybe you take baby steps toward having your own business. Keep your "day job" and pursue your passion as a profession in your own time. Let's say you're an artist and you want to sell your prints. Can you draw or paint on the weekends or at night and set up a shop on Etsy? (I'm sure you know about Etsy. It's the online marketplace where more than $100 million in goods, many of them handmade, are sold each month. The site also receives more than one billion page views monthly, which translates to a lot of eyeballs!)

Maybe you want to open a bakery, but you just can't raise the money. What about street fairs or food fairs on the weekend? They're almost like incubators for small business owners. Or maybe you want to have a vintage-clothing shop. Some boutiques start on eBay before opening physical locations. You still have to pay fees, but it's much, much cheaper than rent and utilities.

What if part-time isn't an option and you need cold, hard cash to get your venture off the ground? Where do you turn? You could borrow money from a bank, friends, family, or investors. Borrowing money from a bank is difficult if you don't have anything to use as collateral, such as real estate. Borrowing money from people you know can be very tricky too, so make sure everyone involved has clear expectations.

There's another option that's wildly popular today—crowdfunding! This is where you get a whole range of people, including strangers, to back your project, business, or idea. The "crowd" literally "funds" it. Have you heard of Kickstarter.com? Kickstarter is the most successful (and legitimate) of all the crowdfunding websites that have sprung up over the past few years. You submit your project to Kickstarter, and if it's approved, your project page goes live on the website. You choose the amount of money you want to raise and give yourself a deadline. If you find enough backers by the deadline, you receive all the money. If you don't, even if you're within a dollar of your goal, you don't receive a dime. Ouch!

Where do the backers come from? Well, everywhere! There are people who simply like what Kickstarter represents and enjoy helping to fund interesting projects. Friends and family members often donate. If you're really ambitious and get press for your project and work social media really hard, you'll get backers that way too.

Now, this isn't free money. As part of the Kickstarter rules, you need to offer something to your backers in exchange. Let's say your Kickstarter project is recording an album of your music and having an actual vinyl album pressed. It's going to cost you $5,000 to record the album, create the physical album, print the album cover, and have the finished product shipped to your apartment. So you set $5,000 as your goal. Maybe anyone who donates $5 will get a pin with your band's name on it; donors at the $25 level get the album; for $250, they get the pin, the album, a poster, and an invitation to the album launch concert; and for $5,000, they get a private concert for their friends. (Dream big!)

If your project is successfully funded, you need to make good on the rewards—or risk a lifetime of bad karma! That means packing everything and schlepping it all to the post office and answering all the e-mails when things are lost in the mail. That in itself can become a full-time job, albeit temporarily.

If you're not familiar with Kickstarter, visit the website and look around. You'll be amazed at the variety of projects. Keep in mind that, Kickstarter has lots of rules and regulations and they don't accept every single project. But if you have something you want to create, Kickstarter could be the perfect way to get your project or business off the ground.

WRITING A BUSINESS PLAN

If you want to start a company, big or small, you need a business plan. Sure, plenty of businesses have gotten off the ground without one, but if you are serious about making a go of your idea, a business plan will help you focus and build a road map of sorts.

Basically, a business plan is an outline of the who, what, where, when, why, and how. What is your business? Who is the customer? Where is the company based? What do you stand for? How will you make money? In your business plan, you figure out what you are selling, making, or doing and project sales and expenses. It can be as elaborate or as simple as you want. If you have no idea where to start, the U.S. Small Business Administration's website (SBA.gov) has a thorough section on how to create a business plan. The entire website, in fact, is very useful for new entrepreneurs.

Don't keep your business plan to yourself. Show a trusted friend, family member, or colleague and ask for feedback. Sometimes you need a second party to poke holes in your proposition and ask questions you might not have considered. You could be so focused that you can't see what an outsider can!

There's a second element to your business plan that I want you to work on. It's your destination. What is that exactly? It's where you want this business to take you. You need to look into the future and really dig deep. It's not enough just to say you want your own business. You can't fly somewhere unless you know where you are going. Having a destination makes the road map more obvious. The vehicle that will get you there is you (and your team if you have one), and the fuel is your motivation.

If you have a business partner, you should discuss the destination together. But if it's just you, you don't need to share the destination with anyone. As long as you know where you're going, that's all that matters.

GET THE BASICS IN PLACE

To get a business going, you need some essentials. Here is a checklist:

- A good name: You need a solid, unique, memorable name for your business. Google the name you would like to use and see what comes up. Make sure no one else is using it. Check social media too. If someone else is using "your" name, think of a new one. Have a brainstorming session with yourself. Get a pen and a piece of paper. Start thinking about your business. What names or words come to mind? Write them down. Go to a thesaurus website and look up synonyms. Go to a dictionary website and start reading words. Write down every word that appeals to you. Still stumped? Start reading song lyrics and poems. Just immerse yourself in words. Once you have a list, decide what your favorites are.

  Be careful of names that are too generic. Your potential customers will have a tough time finding you on the Internet and on social media. If you want to trademark the name, visit the website of the United States Patent and Trademark Office (USPTO.gov). The site features a wealth of information on intellectual property (known as IP) and trademark registration. It's a complicated process. Some businesses hire an IP lawyer if they have the money, but you can do it yourself too. When you search for the name you want to use, you might discover that someone has registered it already. If so, you need another name.

- Branding: I'm talking about your logo, the fonts you use, and the colors that represent your brand. Sometimes these things are called "brand codes." Not every brand needs a logo, but you should pick a font or fonts that represent your brand and use them consistently in correspondence, on social media, and on any packaging. The same goes for colors. If you had to pick two colors, what would they be and why? This kind of consistency conveys a nice level of professionalism, an important thing to communicate when you are a small business.

- Domain name: You need to secure a domain name for your website. A domain name is your basic Web address (for example, www.michellephan.com). Working with a domain registrar, such as Go Daddy, will cost you money, but it's not crazy expensive and there's no way around it. You can register the name for one year or multiple years and buy branded e-mail addresses if you want. If you're trying to save money, use a free, reputable e-mail service instead, such as Google's Gmail. What if your domain name or e-mail address is taken? Again, come up with a new name. Keep it short and simple. You want something your potential customers will remember and find easily.

- Website: You've got your domain name, so now you need a website. You're going to

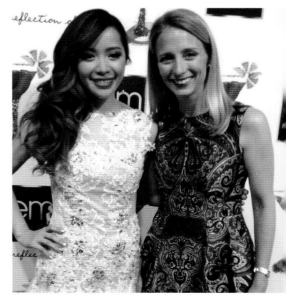

With Jennifer Goldfarb, President of ipsy, at em by Michelle Phan Launch Party.

have one, right? You really cannot have a business today without a website. If you can't afford to have someone design and build one for you, there are plenty of sites available that let you create your own for free! You can start a WordPress blog and use that as your website, or use Facebook. Make sure your website has all your basic information on the homepage. Be sure to include your hours, phone number, e-mail address, and full address. (I've seen addresses on websites that don't include the town, city, or state. How am I supposed to find you?)

- Business cards: Aren't business cards super old-fashioned? Why would you need them? Trust me when I say business cards are the easiest way to make sure someone remembers you and your company. If you bump into a potential customer on the street, in

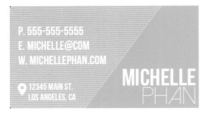

the grocery store, or at a conference, you will want a business card at the ready. Not everyone has the time to stand there and type your info into a smart-phone! Plus, a nicely designed card can communicate a lot about your business and your style.

Business cards don't have to be a big expense. Go online and shop around. Make sure your card contains all the pertinent information—your name, business name, address, phone number, and e-mail. Including your social media handle is a great modern touch. Speaking of which . . .

- Social media: We're going to save this for the next section because a good social media strategy can mean the difference between success and failure for a new entrepreneur. It's that important!

- Licensing and incorporating: Do you need a license for the type of business you want to start? Do you need to incorporate? (To incorporate means to become a corporation. To be an official business in the United States, you need to incorporate.) Don't worry if this sounds scary and complicated! Just Google the words "start a business in" and the name of the state you live in to find the official website with information on how to launch a business in that particular state. Start reading! As with trademarks, you can hire a lawyer to help you through this process, but it is possible to do it on your own.

- Taxes: If you start a business, you will most likely have to pay taxes. It's not a bad thing! Look at it as a sign of your success—you're actually making money. Tax codes are complicated and vary from state to state and city to city, so this might be the one place you want to invest in outside help. Find a good, reputable accountant by asking around. Always get references.

- Signage and hours of operation: If you have an actual store or office, do you have good signage that helps potential customers find you? Have you posted your hours of operation? One of the biggest mistakes that new entrepreneurs make is not posting their hours. I can't tell you how many cute stores and interesting restaurants I walk by that don't post their opening and closing times. Hire a sign maker or make your own sign—it's not that hard, even if you're not a crafty person! Design it on your computer, print it out, clip it to cardboard or stiff-stock paper, punch two holes in the top, run string through it, and attach it to a suction cup on the door or window. Easy!

SOCIAL MEDIA SUCCESS!

As I mentioned in the beginning of this chapter, being an entrepreneur is not easy. It's rewarding and challenging, but any self-employed person will tell you it takes a great deal of work just to break even. A large percentage of small businesses fail, many in the first year of operation. Yet this really is the golden age for entrepreneurism. Technology has made it possible for entrepreneurs to do things themselves that previously needed to be outsourced.

Imagine what it was like for my mother when she opened her own small nail salon two decades ago. She put every dime she had into rent, salaries, and supplies. There was no money for advertising in the local paper or printing fliers at the local print shop. Besides, there were no extra employees to distribute the fliers. She had to rely on word of mouth to get any

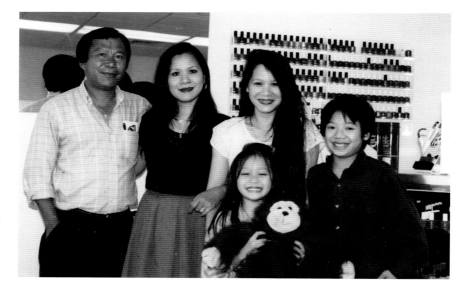

Another fun day at the nail salon with my mom, brother, aunt, and uncle.

business. I can't believe how hard that must have been, just sitting around in her new shop and hoping customers would walk in!

Now imagine if you are opening a nail salon today. You have the entire Internet at your disposal! You can blog, tweet, make videos, e-mail your friends, communicate with beauty bloggers, you name it. You no longer have to wait for people to stumble upon you.

But let's take a step back. Chances are, if you are like most entrepreneurs just starting out, you don't have a lot of people working for you or a social media team. (If you do, congratulations!) You have . . . you. Before you launch your business, you need to have your social media strategy in place. Social media is a gift to all budding entrepreneurs because the cost of entry is truly free, as long as you have access to a computer and an Internet connection. (If you have neither, head to your local public library and use theirs.) You need to showcase your work. You can't grow your business in the dark. You have to shine a light on it for other people to see.

Some small-business people think social media means taking advantage of everything the Internet has to offer. They're making videos for YouTube! They have a Tumblr and a blog! They're tweeting ten times a day! Don't confuse doing *everything* with having a social media strategy. They are two completely different things. One will make you crazy; one could help make you successful.

Here's a checklist to get you started:

- The top platforms: This could change tomorrow, but as of today, the most popular platforms for businesses trying to connect with customers are Facebook, Twitter, YouTube, Google+, Instagram, Foursquare, Yelp, and Tumblr. Of course, there are more, but these eight are the ones you need to know about.

- Claim your name: As I mentioned earlier, your social media strategy will not include posting on every platform in existence. Even the biggest brands in the world focus on a set number of platforms. That said, I want you to claim your name on the major platforms mentioned above. Social media is an ever-changing world. You want to be ready if a certain platform becomes red-hot, and you don't want someone else taking your company name as his or her handle. That does happen! While you're at it, you might as well add your address and hours of operation if that is an option.

- Consistent naming: You want the same name across all platforms. You don't want to be Company ABC on one platform and ABC Co. on another. That will confuse your customers and fans. Find the one name that works across everything.

- Pick your platform: How do you know what platform your business should be on? Which do you already use to communicate with your friends, family members, and current or former classmates? Let's start there—you already have some followers! Those connections will come in handy. When you are an entrepreneur or small-business person, you need your friends and family to help spread the word.

  You also need to consider what platforms are the most beloved or frequented by your customer base. If you're a kids' photographer, don't waste your time on Twitter, which is text based. A more visual medium is better for you, such as Instagram or Facebook. If you have a blog about your neighborhood or industry, then Twitter might be the place for you because it's newsier and immediate and a great place to share links.

  Don't feel you need to go with the most popular platform. Pick the one that has the strongest community that will support your vision.

- Your time investment: This is probably the most important thing you need to consider. How much time can you spend on social media? Don't tell me no time! Social media is key to your potential success. You need to carve out time (preferably daily) to monitor and update. This is why it's best to focus on one or two platforms and commit to doing them well. Robust activity on one site is so much better than halfhearted activity on multiple sites. If you're a total pro at social media and have the time, feel free to post on as many platforms as you think is right for your brand.

  You truly do need to regularly monitor the platform(s) you are on. What if a customer asks a question or has a complaint? You don't want to miss it.

- Creative content: To be truly successful on social media, you need fans and followers. Otherwise, you're just talking to yourself! So how do you get lots of followers? Hold on! We're getting ahead of ourselves here. Before you can get followers, you need to decide what kind of content you are going to post.

  You need interesting content that entertains or informs—preferably both. You want people to look forward to your posts and come back for more. People want to follow you. They want to hear your words and see your vision.

  Once you decide what you would like to post, you need to decide when you are going to post and how often. It's not dissimilar to your personal social media presence. You should never post so frequently that it becomes annoying. Another thing to consider is posting different kinds of content on different days.

  Whatever you decide, you need to plan all of this in advance. Otherwise, you'll be making up your social media strategy as you go.

  Put together a schedule of what and when and post accordingly. This also means creating your content in advance. Now, if you have a coffee shop or food truck with a new special each day, you'll need to do some more last-minute posting. But you will still find it helpful to bank a number of photos, videos, or links in advance so you aren't constantly scrambling for new content. Investigate such online tools as HootSuite or TweetDeck, which allow

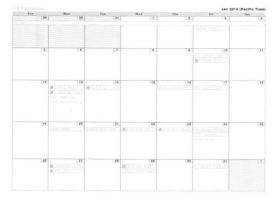

you to post in advance as well as monitor multiple platforms.

Stick to your schedule, but don't be afraid to adapt or shift based on current events or the natural evolution of your business. It's like your business plan. What worked in the beginning might not work three months or a year from now. Being nimble is part of being a smart business-person, but so is staying the course. You need to find a balance.

Still confused about or unsure what is best regarding social media? Take a look at what your competitors are doing. Don't steal from them. That's not cool. But you can certainly learn best practices or get inspiration from the leaders in your field.

- Fans and followers: If you're lucky, people will find you, but usually you need to go find them. Part of having a social media strategy is being smart about whom you follow. Ask yourself who is important to your company or brand. Figure out who needs to know you exist. Are there editors or bloggers key to your industry? Neighborhood groups or businesses? Stylists or makeup artists? Live music venues?

  And don't overlook friends, family members, colleagues, and classmates. Hopefully, they'll be happy to follow your business and even promote it to their circles. Send a nice e-mail asking them to follow your new enterprise and spread the word. It can be a mass e-mail; just remember to BCC everyone rather than CC. CCing is never good. Some people like to keep their e-mail addresses private and avoid sharing it with strangers.

  Do you need to follow everyone who follows you? Not necessarily. If you want to convey that you're nice and friendly, perhaps that is the way to go. But maybe you want to convey a sense of exclusivity and only follow tastemakers. That's okay too.

  You've followed people, you've been strategic about it, and still nothing? Let's buckle down. Now you need to . . .

- Engage: Don't despair if no one is commenting, liking, or retweeting. Part of being successful on social media is engaging with others. That old saying "If you build it, they will come" doesn't apply to social media. You need to be, well, *social* and put out that virtual welcome mat! Are you retweeting, leaving comments for, and liking the right people? If you're a jewelry designer and there's a fashion magazine stylist whose work you love, tell him or her! "Loved your tribal story in the new *Elle!*" Are you a makeup artist and want to work with a specific photographer? Comment on his or her Instagram photos. Get a dialogue going. Get on his or her radar.

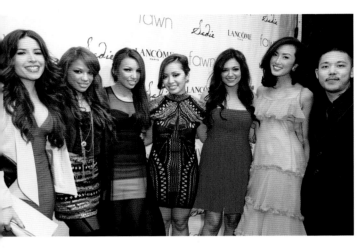

On the red carpet at the FAWN launch party.

If you already have some suppliers (meaning other companies you pay to supply you with things you need) or distributors (meaning boutiques, stores, e-tailers, etc., that carry your product or do business with you), create some posts that mention them by name. Make sure to tag them correctly. Chances are, they will follow you and retweet, like, or comment. The better you do, the better they do, so it's in everyone's best interest to help one another.

Perhaps you need to join a forum or attend some conferences. Investigate those options. You need to get yourself out there, in life and online. No one is going to know about you unless you speak up! Networking still doesn't come easy to me. In the beginning of my career, I went to lots of events, even though it was my least favorite thing to do. I just wanted to be home editing my tutorials or playing video games. But I did wind up meeting some amazing people, many of whom were very helpful to my career. Connections matter.

CUSTOMER DATABASE

Once you start getting customers, you want to keep track of them and communicate with them. Give some thought to how you will collect contact information. Is there a sign-up option on your website? Is there a notebook or sign-up sheet in your store/gallery/salon/booth where guests can leave their names? What do you plan to do with those names?

There are several marketing/e-mail services available today, such as Constant Contact, MyEmma, and MailChimp, that make it easy to keep track of your customers' e-mails and to create engaging e-mail campaigns to send to your database. These aren't free, but they will make your life easier if you have hundreds of e-mail addresses to monitor and keep track of. Also, it's easy for customers to opt out of getting your e-mails, which is important because you never want to aggravate a potential or current client. Speaking of which . . .

GOOD CUSTOMER SERVICE

If you have customers, clients, or guests, you want to be focused on providing good customer service. It's a great reputation to have. If anyone has a complaint or problem with your business, you should deal with it as fast as possible. Otherwise, you know what could happen. He or she could post something on Twitter or Yelp—or, worse, get in touch with the Better Business Bureau with a complaint about you. Own up to whatever you did wrong and fix the problem.

Sometimes the customer is in the wrong, but you still need to be nice and resolve the issue. Don't ever pick a fight with a customer or client. That is a recipe for disaster! If someone posts on social media, don't respond point by point. It's always a shock when someone complains about you or your business so publicly, but simply say, "Hi, [name of person]. Please e-mail me at [fill in your e-mail] and we'll certainly resolve this. Thank you." Take the conversation out of the public space. I've made the mistake of responding publicly in the past and I learned how things can be misunderstood, so now I follow this advice!

HOW TO DO PUBLIC RELATIONS

Public relations is a practice in which you get information about your business out to the public, mainly through the media. With public relations, you reach out to those who can write about or feature your business in some way. You don't pay to be featured. Any time you pay, that is either advertising or sponsored content.

Here's how to get started:

- Decide what you are promoting: Promote just one thing at a time. If you have ten new products, that's too much. Pick one product or one event. Or maybe your business is brand new. That counts as your one thing!

- Write a press release: A press release doesn't have to be long at all. In fact, it should be one page or even shorter. Describe your company or brand and what it is you are promoting. Be sure to include why it is new and noteworthy. Don't waste anyone's time with old news. Include a quote from yourself and/or another party involved in the project. Include all the particulars: address, hours, prices, launch date, etc. Put a headline on it and include your contact information.

- Put a media list together: Who could potentially write about your company or product? We'd all love to see our companies in *Time* or *People* or on CNN, but that probably isn't realistic just yet! Let's take it down a notch and focus on local media. Find any blogs, magazines, newspapers, websites, or TV shows that cover your town, city, or region. Check them out and see who writes about what. If you're pitching a story on something fashion related, you don't want to send it to the person who writes about food! Find the right names and see if there are e-mail addresses or contact information listed anywhere. If not, try Twitter. You can tweet at the publication/blog/website/etc., and say, "Hi there. I'd like to send an e-mail to [person or publication name]. What's the best way to get in touch?"

When you write to that person, send a very short, specific

e-mail. Identify who you are and say that you are writing because you would love for him or her to consider covering your company/project/product/event/etc. Attach the press release, proofread, and hit send. Now, he or she may not write back to you. As I've said before, don't become a stalker! Members of the media get pitches all day long, so they might be too busy to write back. Or perhaps what you sent isn't of interest to them. If you don't hear back for several days, you can write one more time, but that's it. Try forwarding the original message and write, "Just checking in on this. Would love to discuss with you." Or something to that effect. If that doesn't elicit a response, move on to the next person. You always can circle back to the original person when you have something else to promote.

Let's say you want to pitch something to the national media—say, a major magazine such as *Bazaar* or *GQ* or a website such as Refinery29. Go for it! It's great that you're thinking big. The national media writes about newcomers all the time, and you might be just the newcomer they're looking for. But again, don't be disappointed if you don't hear back. The best entrepreneurs learn to deal with rejection and not take it personally.

- Photos/samples/invitations: Once you send your e-mail with the press release attached, you might get a response. If the recipient is interested in covering your business, he or she might ask for a few extras, such as photos. Do you have photos to go along with the story? It's always a smart idea to have good pictures of yourself and the other people involved in your business, as well as pictures of any physical location and/or products you offer. Let's say you and your best friend sell gluten-free cookies and cupcakes at a local flea market and you have a very cool new flavor you think will rock the world. You should have pictures of the two of you, both posed and in action; pictures of your booth at the market; and pictures of the products you sell. If you don't have the money for professional photographs, get a friend to take some good pictures. Smartphones make it easier than ever to take quality photos.

What if the writer/blogger/editor wants to try your product?

Or what if he or she wants to borrow it to photograph it? Make sure you're prepared to respond. How will you get him or her the cupcake, or the piece of jewelry, or whatever it is that you are promoting? Last, if you're having an event, do you invite the writer/blogger/editor? It's entirely up to you and it depends on how exclusive the event is.

• Success: Someone featured you in a blog post or article! Congratulations! Make sure to thank whoever was behind it. Sending a gift is a bit over the top, but a nicely written e-mail is perfect. Then make sure to put the article, blog post, video, whatever it is, on your social media and include the handles for the writer/editor/blogger and the media outlet.

Whether social media or traditional media, it's all about spreading the word and being an evangelist for your business.

BE COLLABORATIVE

Just a quick word about collaborations. So many companies do special partnerships today. Look at everything Target, H&M, and MAC do with outside partners. Yes, they are giant companies, but you can do it too! It's a modern way to stay fresh, be creative, and expand your customer base. Be on the lookout for other start-ups and entrepreneurs you can partner with on products, events, videos—you name it. You don't have to be in the same place to collaborate. You can partner with someone halfway around the world and do something online together.

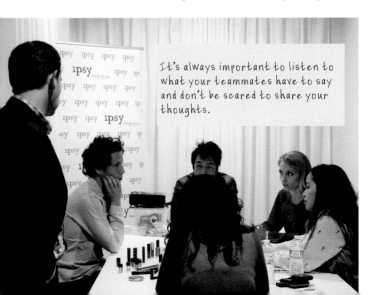

It's always important to listen to what your teammates have to say and don't be scared to share your thoughts.

HOW TO BE A BOSS

Many people become entrepreneurs because they want to be their own boss. Often, however, that comes with being someone else's boss. You don't always think about that part. Are you prepared to be the person in charge? It's not always fun. Becoming a boss and thinking like one has certainly been a big challenge for me. It's a hard role to fill, especially if you have no prior experience managing people or leading a team. Many people have the wrong idea about what it means to be the boss. They think you have to be mean and crack the whip all the time. They rule by fear. I believe that nurturing and empowering your team members is a better way to go. Being kind doesn't mean you're weak!

The hardest part of being the boss is firing people. I hate it. It's like a relationship in that there's no easy way to break up with someone. Be quick, honest, and direct with the person you are letting go. I wish I had advice on how to make it easier, but I don't.

The last thing to keep in mind about being the boss involves working with friends. If you can avoid it, avoid it! I've seen too many friendships go sour over a start-up. But if you want to work with your bestie, there are ways to make it a success. Make sure to have some honest conversations in the beginning, especially about money. Decide up front who takes care of what tasks. If you are equal partners, decide how you're dividing the various responsibilities and the decision making.

DON'T BE AFRAID OF FAILURE

These are my final words of entrepreneurial advice: Be fearless! It's a tough world out there and it's going to take everything you have to make it work.

If this path takes you down a road you didn't expect, that's okay. Life is like that sometimes. But I know that along the way you'll meet interesting people and learn some major lessons—about work, life, and most important, yourself.

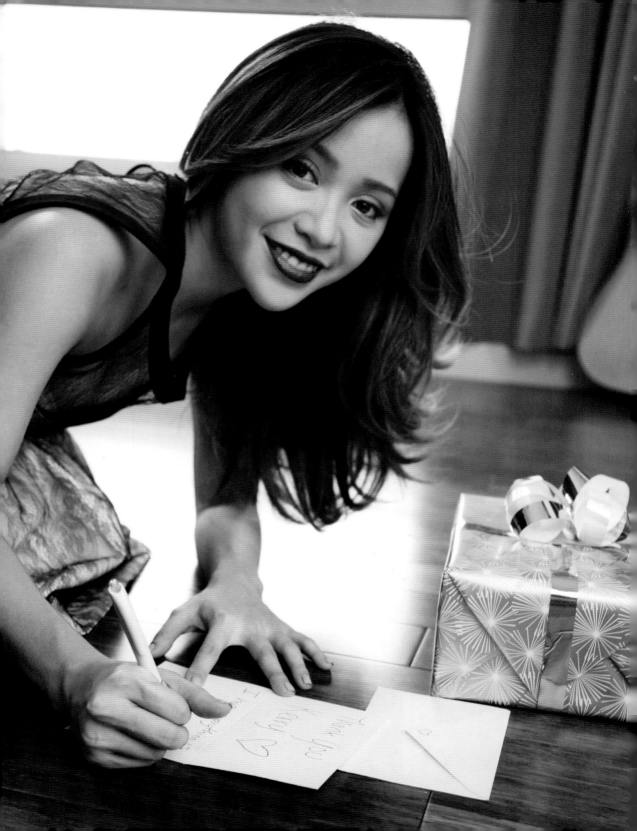

MODERN MANNERS MADE EASY

Everyone knows what the word *manners* means, right? It's forms of behavior that convey respect for other people. Some might use the term *etiquette*. Whichever word you prefer, they both describe what we'll be talking about in this chapter. Manners and etiquette might seem like fussy, old-fashioned things to talk about, but think about it. Manners are what keep civilization civilized. Having rules for how to act and conduct ourselves can make life easier and smoother. Rather than wondering what to do in certain situations, those rules let us know exactly what to do.

Etiquette is a bit of a lost art today, but I'm going to help you understand what you need to know and why, and for what situations. We're not going to talk about fish forks and how to curtsy. That's a bit advanced, and unless you're a member of a royal family somewhere, you don't really need to know that. Instead, I'm going to focus on situations that you will probably encounter as you go about your normal life.

Manners really aren't any different from makeup, skin care, or fashion, come to think of it. They're all things that help us present our best selves to the world around us.

MY TWO BIG RULES

I have two major rules when it comes to manners that you can apply to every single situation without fail. The first is that you need to have situational awareness. That simply means taking in the environment around you and quickly processing the rules of behavior for that situation. Here's one example. Today's the first day of your new job. You walk in the office and quickly scan the surroundings. Let's say it is an open-plan setting with lots of low cubicles and no offices. What are people wearing? How loudly are the employees talking, both on the phone and to each other? Is the office very social and bustling, or do people just go about their business quietly? Is anyone wearing headphones and listening to music as they work? Do people eat at their desks?

You figure out the answers on your own and immediately apply them to your own behavior. If no one is drinking coffee at his or her desk, don't plop your grande Frappuccino next to your computer. Finish it in the kitchen. If everyone works quietly, don't call your BFF and detail every last thing about last night's date so your officemates can hear. Send her a text and fill her in during your lunch break. See how this works? It's about taking off your blinders and observing how other people act in a certain situation. You can learn a lot when you are observant. This isn't just for work—it applies to school, parties, the subway, almost any scenario. Sometimes the rules of behavior are right in front of us. We just need to take the time to see them.

Some people are blessed with great situational awareness; others need to work at it or be told what the exact rules of behavior are. The good news is that it is like a muscle you can strengthen with a little bit of work. You just need to be mindful and remember to look around and assess. With a little practice, you will get better at it. I promise.

My second rule is to respect everyone. Older, younger—it doesn't matter. I'm sure you want to be treated with respect, so give everyone else that courtesy.

I really believe that if you practice situational awareness and treat everyone with respect, you will be okay no matter where you go or what you do. A decent person who pays attention and treats others well? That's modern manners right there.

Now, about that fork . . .

AT THE TABLE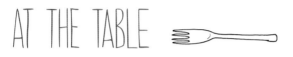

Mealtime is when you really need good manners. Whether it's a date or a business luncheon, you don't want to be the person who doesn't know which bread plate or glass is yours. That is definitely embarrassing. So let's review some dining basics. None of this is too tricky or complicated, or will make you look like a snob. You'll just seem smart and polite.

Here are a few helpful tips:

- When you sit down, put your napkin in your lap. If you need to leave the table at any point during the meal, you can fold your napkin and place it to the left of your plate or on your chair. If you have a big red lipstick smear or something else obvious on the napkin, fold it so that the other guests don't see that.

- If you don't know the other people at the table, make sure to introduce yourself. Just tell them your name. You don't need to tell them your life story.

- Put your phone away in your bag or coat pocket. Do not put it on the table.

- Do not put your elbows on the table.

- Sit up straight. Definitely don't hunch over your food like a caveman protecting his meal.

- Chew with your mouth closed.

- Don't talk with your mouth full.

- Don't ever put your napkin on top of your plate, even when you are finished.

- When cutting your food, cut one bite at a time. Don't cut your entire steak or pork chop into pieces and then proceed to eat each little piece.

THE PROPER PLACE SETTING

Whether you are setting a table or sitting at one, here is a guide to what goes where:

If there are multiple courses of food being served, use your utensils in the order they are placed on the table, from the outside in. Your fork or forks will be on the left. The smaller fork, on the outside, is for salad or

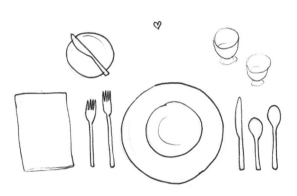

appetizers. The larger fork is for the main course. On the right are your knife (sharp side facing the plate) and spoon(s). If soup is being served, the soup spoon will be on the outside, followed sometimes by a dessert spoon. Other times, the utensils for dessert could be placed horizontally at the top of your plate.

Your bread plate will always be to the left of your plate and silverware. Your glasses will always be to the right.

If you are in the middle of your meal and need to pause to talk—or maybe run to the bathroom—leave your utensils on your plate, in an inverted V-shape, with the tines of the fork touching the knife. When you're finished eating, put your utensils parallel, fork on the left, knife on the right, and the knife's edge facing the fork. This signals that you are done.

WHAT DID I JUST BITE INTO?

Sometimes during the course of a meal, you bite into something unpleasant. Maybe it's a pit, a fish bone, or a bit of gristle. What do you do? Well, don't panic or get embarrassed. You didn't do anything wrong! It just happens sometimes. If you can remove the item from your mouth with a fork, go ahead and put it on the side of your plate. If it's a pit or a bone, use your fingers or your napkins and again, put it on your plate. Just don't make a big production of it or hide the item in your napkin. That just looks weird and makes it more obvious. The cooler you seem about the situation, the less anyone will care.

If olives have been placed on the table for you to snack on, the host or the restaurant usually provides a bowl in which you can place the pits. If not, just put them on your plate. It's okay to remove them from your mouth with your fingers. Just remember to wipe your fingers on your napkin.

These rules only apply to inedible things. If you've bitten into something you don't like, well, that's too bad. You have to eat it. Don't spit it into your napkin and hide it, and don't ever spit it directly onto your plate. Just be a big boy or girl and eat your food. It won't kill you.

Now, if you have an allergy or a certain diet—say, you're allergic to peanuts and/or a vegan—you need to communicate that as early as possible. If you're attending an event, tell the host or organizer about any dietary needs in advance. If you're at a restaurant, let the server know when he or she hands you the menu. Just say, "I'm [fill in the blank about your food issue], is there anything I should avoid?"

Does a guy need to stand up if a woman leaves the table?
It's polite but not always necessary. It used to be an ironclad etiquette rule, the same as holding open doors for women and having men go first in revolving doors (the thought being that the first person would do most of the heavy pushing). It's nice for a guy to be a gentleman and do those things from time to time, but no one will judge him if he doesn't. That said, whether you're a man or a woman, it's always polite to hold doors open.

DIGITAL GADGETS AT THE TABLE

Oh, boy. This is a controversial subject. Some restaurants prohibit the use of phones in the dining room. This means no checking e-mail, photographing your food, or texting your friends. If you need to use the phone, you are expected to go outside, or perhaps into the hall. If those are the restaurant's rules, you need to follow them.

But what if there's nothing posted on the menu, or you're at a private event or someone's home? Well, then you should use your common sense and good judgment. I think it's always good to put your phone away and not leave it resting on the table. Just practically speaking, what if someone spills a glass of water or some other liquid on the table? You'll be glad that your phone is tucked away in your handbag! Also, phones on the table make it too convenient to look at the screen. Let's say you pick up your phone and take a quick look. Next thing you know, everyone is looking at his or her phone, the conversation has died, and you become one of those tables where the guests are more interested in their e-mail than one another. That's always kind of sad. So rise above the temptation and focus on your friends and the food.

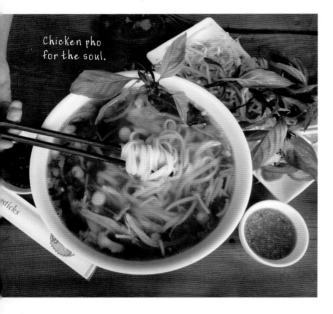

Chicken pho for the soul.

As for the food, is it okay to take pictures and post them to your social media outlets? Again, it depends. Is it a really nice restaurant where this kind of thing is frowned upon? Then it's probably best to leave your phone in your bag until you are finished. Is it a fun, buzzy restaurant that just served you the coolest-looking appetizer ever? Go ahead and take a picture then. But don't spend more time photographing the food than *enjoying* the food. That's boring for your tablemates. You also don't need to provide the world with real-time running commentary of your meal. You always can post pictures *after* your meal.

Be careful about using a flash in a restaurant. You never want to disturb the guests around you. If it's too dark, so be it. The planet won't stop spinning because people couldn't see your awesome plate of sushi. If you really want to take the picture and it's dark, hold a candle close to the food to light it.

Situational awareness definitely comes into play in these cases. Look around and see what's going on in the restaurant. Figure out what behavior is welcome or not welcome and act accordingly.

What about tablets? They don't really have a place at the table when you're dining with guests. They're way too big and obtrusive to use for photos. But if you're eating by yourself and you'd like to read on your tablet, go ahead. It's no different from reading a book or a magazine when dining solo.

YOU ARE INVITED TO A PARTY

That's nice! Someone is having a special event and they want you to come. Chances are you were invited a) in person, b) via e-mail or text, or c) with a printed invitation. The first thing you need to do is RSVP, which means accept or decline the invitation. What does *RSVP* mean exactly? It's French for "*répondez s'il vous plaît.*" (You pronounce it "ray-pon-day see voo play.") In English, that means "respond, please." So you RSVP either yes or no. It's rude not to RSVP, even if the invitation was casual. If someone is nice enough to invite you somewhere or to something, you should have the courtesy to let him or her know your intentions. It's frustrating to throw a party and not know who is attending. It's nice to RSVP as soon as you can. Don't wait until the last minute.

WHAT IS THE DRESS CODE?

Dress code? What's that, you ask? It's a suggestion from the host about what you should (or in some cases, what you are expected to) wear. Here are some dress codes you might see on an invitation:

Black tie: This means the men and women should dress in formal attire. It's called black tie because it used to be that black bow ties, worn with tuxedos, were a must for the male guests in this case. Nowadays, there is more flexibility, but you are still expected to be very dressed up. No jeans, flip-flops, or day wear of any kind should be worn. Unless you are incredibly confident in your fashion choices and have a very specific look you are famous for, you'll be embarrassed if you show up in casual clothing. If you don't own any formal attire, don't panic. Rent, borrow, or hit a vintage store and find something you can afford. For men, a plain black suit with a simple black tie always looks classic. Women can never go wrong with a simple but elegant black dress. You can also transform a basic dress into something formal with the right accessories.

(White tie is similar in that it's formal, but the men are expected to wear white bow ties with their tuxedos instead of black ones.)

Festive: What in the world does *festive* mean? It means what it says. Wear something fun! It's less formal than black tie, but you're still expected to put some effort into it. If your idea of festive is your pajamas, that's not what we're talking about here. Wear something dressy and celebratory. Think colorful, sparkly, or shiny. Don't dress like a wallflower.

Casual: This means you can wear jeans, daytime clothing, or work attire, but you should still look nice. You're going to an event, after all. Don't dress like you just rolled out of bed.

Business casual: This means you need to look nice and professional, but you can be slightly relaxed about it. No suits or stuffy attire.

Cocktail attire: Think of this as girls'-night-out clothes. You can wear trendy outfits, from dresses to blouses with cute pants.

Come as you are: Yes, this is an actual dress code. This means come however you like. If you're the kind of girl who gets dressed up all the time, then dress up! If you always rock a hoodie and your old Nikes, wear those. No one will judge you—or at least they shouldn't.

WHAT IS A HOSTESS GIFT?

Sometimes, you're expected to bring a gift to an event. If it's a birthday party or a wedding or something similar, you should definitely give a gift. If it's a housewarming party or a dinner party, it's always thoughtful to bring a little something. That's called a hostess gift (even if the hostess is a he!). This doesn't have to be anything elaborate. It can be a nice scented candle, a book, or some chocolates. The host or hostess is under no obligation to share the gift with the guests, so don't be offended if he or she doesn't offer you any of the chocolates!

Flowers are always lovely too, but they aren't a great hostess gift. Why? Well, the host or hostess is probably busy getting everything ready and he or she will have to stop what they're doing, find something to put the flowers in, and then find somewhere to put them.

But truly, any kind of gift is lovely. As they say, it's the thought that counts!

THANK-YOU NOTES AND E-MAILS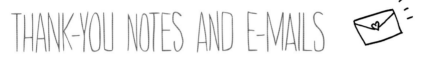

The day after the party, send a written note or an e-mail. (A text is okay too. It's better than nothing!) Hosts and hostesses like to know that their guests had a great time, so be sure to say thank you and mention a highlight or two. Nothing's a bigger bummer than throwing a party and not hearing from anyone the next day. If you attended a wedding, you're not expected to send a note, but I'm sure the bride and groom will be thrilled to hear from you. Just a text message is nice, since they're probably en route to their honeymoon.

HOW TO WRITE A THANK-YOU NOTE

If you've never written a proper thank-you note before, it's simple. Just be sincere, thank the gift giver for the specific item he or she gave you, and mention why you like it. You don't have to write a novel! Here's an example:

Dear Kate,

It was so nice of you to remember how much I love Georgia O'Keeffe's work! Thank you for the beautiful art book. I already have it displayed in my living room. My sister has tried to steal it twice!!

XOXO,
Mish

You can certainly send a thank-you via e-mail, but a handwritten thank-you note is very special. The most important thing is that you send something. A fun gesture these days is to text a picture of you with the gift to the gift giver. Don't forget to include a sentence actually saying thank you. At the very least, it's important to acknowledge that you received the gift, especially if someone sent it to you in the mail! That way, he or she won't worry about whether the gift actually arrived.

HOW TO WRITE A CONDOLENCE NOTE

There are going to be times in your life when you have to write a difficult note to a friend or family member. Perhaps someone has died or is ill and you want to show your support or concern or offer your condolences. The recipient of your note will appreciate that you care. Share a special anecdote or memory if you have one. If not, be brief and sincere. Here is an example:

> Dear James,
>
> I'm so sorry to hear that your grandmother passed away. I still remember all those times she made us dinner when we were in grammar school. I know how much you and your brother loved her. My sincerest condolences to your family and please know you are in my thoughts.
>
> Love,
> Michelle

Again, it's a nice gesture to send this as a handwritten note. A human touch is very special. But e-mail is okay too. The most important thing is just sending a message.

HOW TO MAKE EYE CONTACT

I find a lot of people don't understand how to make eye contact these days. Could it be all the time spent on the Internet? Or texting? Whatever the reason, it's hard to be taken seriously when you can't look someone in the eye. If I'm talking to someone, I want him or her to acknowledge me. I need to see that someone is listening and paying attention to what I'm saying. It's especially important in a work context. When you're talking to your boss or a colleague, you don't want to stare at the floor or the wall the whole time.

As I explained in the chapter on finding and keeping a job, you should look someone in the eye as he or she talks to you. Now, it's okay to break eye contact every now and then. It's a little mental or conversation break. You just kind of pause and rethink and bring your gaze back to the person in front of you. You don't want to overstare, because it can make the other person feel uncomfortable.

HOW TO SHAKE HANDS

As I also explained in the jobs chapter, a good handshake is essential in life. When you shake hands with someone you've just met, you don't want him or her to think anything except that it was nice meeting you. If he or she walks away thinking, "Wow, he/she almost broke my hand," or "That person had the weakest handshake ever," you didn't make a good first impression.

It's easy to practice a good handshake with a friend or family member. Shake hands with him or her and ask what he or she thinks. You want to gently grasp the other person's hand and actually shake it (that's why it's called a handshake!), but in a controlled upward manner. Don't put your hand in the other person's like it is a dead fish and make him or her do all the work. And don't crush his or her hand like you're the Incredible Hulk.

You might be thinking, "Michelle, you don't have to tell me how to shake someone's hand!" But trust me. There are lots of people with terrible hand-shakes who don't know it. It's an easy thing to fix, so it's good to find out where you stand.

HOW TO MAKE CONVERSATION

The last thing we're going to talk about in this chapter is how to be a good conversationalist. What does this have to do with manners or etiquette? Everything! If you have a hard time talking to others, you could be written off as rude. Maybe that's not the case at all and you're just shy. Or you get tongue-tied around people you don't know. That's okay. I know what it's like to be shy. I was an introvert for years. But part of life is knowing how to hold your own in social situations, so you need to be prepared.

Believe it or not, it's not that hard to make conversation. There are a few questions you should have tucked in the back of your mind that you can pull out at any time.

- Where are you from?
- What brings you here?
- How do you know [mutual friend's name]?
- What do you study at school?
- Where do you work?

A good thing to remember is to ask questions that start with inter-rogative words, such as *who, what, where, why, when,* and *how.* If you ask questions that can be answered with a yes or a no, your conversation might not go very far. Think "How long have you lived here?" or "How do you like living here?" versus "Do you live here?" If you know the person al-ready, ask what his or her plans are for the holiday or a simple "What have you been up to?"

Also, you need to be mindful of with whom you are speaking. If some-one is older than you or more senior than you, be respectful. Don't speak to them in the casual tone you would use to talk to your friends. It might seem funny to you, but it can be taken as a form of disrespect. So no *yo, bro, hey,* or *wassup.*

SET WITH ETIQUETTE

Mind your manners? No problem. Now you can feel comfortable in a whole range of social settings and situations. At the end of the day, so much of life is about having respect for others and respect for yourself. Manners aren't meant to change your personality or hide what you're all about. They're a tool, like your laptop and your lipstick. When used correctly, they can make your life a whole lot better.

ASK MICHELLE

Sometimes, it's the little things that reveal a lot about a person. Here are a few facts about me that I thought you might find interesting. How would you answer these questions? And do you know how your friends and family would answer? Maybe it would be fun to ask them.

What color makes you the happiest?
Sunshine yellow

What movie do you watch over and over?
Spirited Away

Who inspires you?
My mother, teachers, nurses, children, Princess Diana, Bruce Lee, Banksy, and Bob Marley

What book do you love?
The Bible and *The Giving Tree*

What music do you listen to the most?
Bob Marley, Journey, Whitney Houston, Nat King Cole, classical, and soundtracks from movies, TV shows, and video games

Who is your favorite fictional character?
Alice from *Alice in Wonderland*

What food can't you live without?
Vietnamese food. Chicken pho in particular.

What is the most amazing place you've visited?
New Zealand. It took my breath away.

What is your favorite museum? The Rodin Museum in Paris

How do you unwind? I throw on my pajamas. That's the moment I can take it easy.

Do you get stressed out?
Yes, but it's good stress!

What is your favorite season?

 Summer. It used to be winter. See how people can change?

Are you a morning person or a night person?

 Naturally, I'm a night person, but I've trained myself to be a morning person.

If you had a superpower, what would it be?

 To have healing powers.

Who is your favorite superhero?

 Batman. He was my first-ever toy figurine before I had a doll.

Do you cook?

 Only for special occasions.

Do you have a sweet tooth?

 Not really, but if something is sweet and salty, yes! Heavenly combination.

What is your favorite flower?

 Lotus

Do you have a motto?

 Live and love freely.

Do you like animals?

 Yes. The cuddlier and fuzzier, the better.

What do you like to do when you have a day off?

 Play video games, catch up on movies and TV shows, and visit museums.

What is your favorite ice cream flavor?

 Vanilla. Plain and simple is always the best.

What is one skill you don't have but wish you did?

 To be good at martial arts.

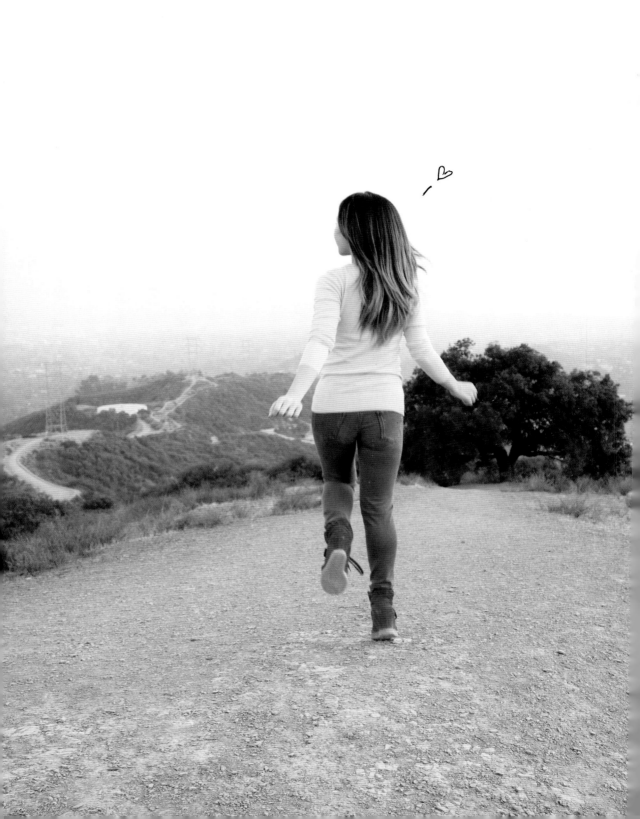

GOOD LUCK!

Well, we're at the end. We made it! Thank you for reading through these pages and taking this trip with me. I hope you found some words of wisdom and learned a few things that will help you on your journey, because your life *is* a journey. But the path is one that you create. We don't need to follow the map that has been handed to us; we can draw our own.

I've never believed in destiny; instead, I'm a big believer in opportunity. Just because you were born to a certain station in life doesn't mean you are stuck there. I'm living proof of that, for sure. Each of us is capable of evolution, change, and greatness.

Maybe for you that means leading a humble, honest life—there is certainly greatness in that. For others, it means being the next Einstein or Steve Jobs. Whatever you pursue, I hope you understand that life is precious. It has nothing to do with acquiring the latest tech gadget, pair of jeans, or handbag, although that stuff can be fun. But don't let it distract you. The important stuff is how you go about each day and how you treat others.

We covered a lot of ground in this book, from my parents to manners to bullying to jobs and internships. Are you ready to take on the world now? I hope so! If I had to summarize everything from the previous chapters and give you an action plan, I would say these three things:

Be kind

Be grateful

Be fearless

If you watch my YouTube tutorials, you know that I end every video with the words *good luck*. Because I take my position as a teacher seriously, I do this as a way to encourage everyone. But luck isn't something I can hand to you or magically convey. You create your own luck. It's not about lying in bed, waiting for something mystical to happen and transform your life. It's about getting out of bed and exploring what the universe has to offer—and what you have to offer in return.

Once you close this book and put it on your shelf or give it to a friend, I want you to go forward and be brave. No matter what comes your way, it will be okay. As my mother once told me, life never puts anything in your path that you can't handle. Happy travels!

♡ Mish

ACKNOWLEDGMENTS

I'd like to thank the following people who inspired this book...

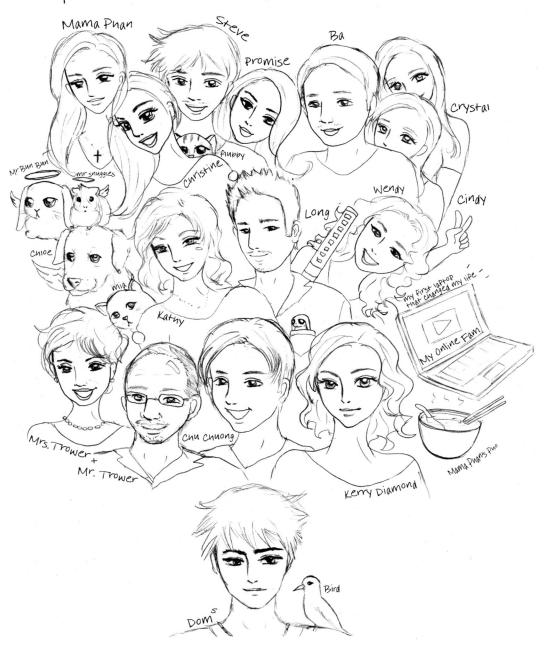

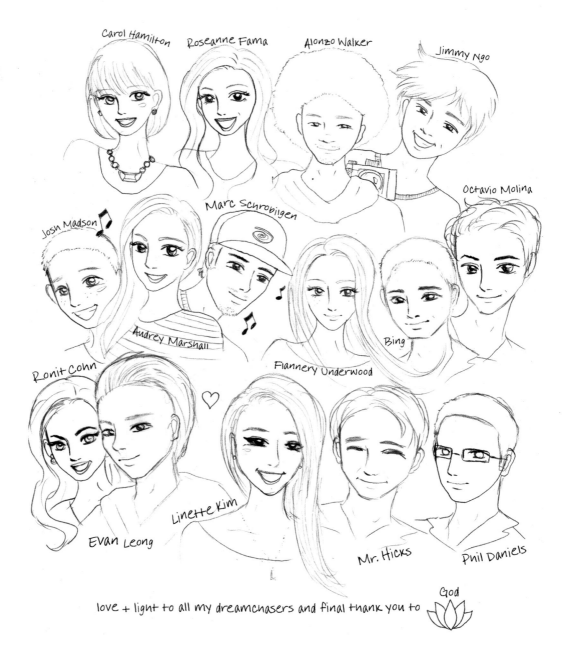

Carol Hamilton

Roseanne Fama

Alonzo Walker

Jimmy Ngo

Octavio Molina

Josh Madson

Marc Schrobilgen

Audrey Marshall

Bing

Ronit Cohn

Flannery Underwood

Evan Leong

Linette Kim

Mr. Hicks

Phil Daniels

love + light to all my dreamchasers and final thank you to God

INDEX